Performer Training
for Actors and Athletes

Performer Training
for Actors and Athletes

Frank Camilleri

methuen | drama

LONDON • NEW YORK • OXFORD • NEW DELHI • SYDNEY

METHUEN DRAMA
Bloomsbury Publishing Plc
50 Bedford Square, London, WC1B 3DP, UK
1385 Broadway, New York, NY 10018, USA
29 Earlsfort Terrace, Dublin 2, Ireland

BLOOMSBURY, METHUEN DRAMA and the Methuen Drama logo
are trademarks of Bloomsbury Publishing Plc

First published in Great Britain 2023

Copyright © Frank Camilleri, 2023

Frank Camilleri has asserted his right under the Copyright, Designs and
Patents Act, 1988, to be identified as author of this work.

For legal purposes the Acknowledgements on p. xxxii constitute
an extension of this copyright page.

Cover design: Ben Anslow
Cover image © Jeremy de Maria

All rights reserved. No part of this publication may be reproduced or transmitted
in any form or by any means, electronic or mechanical, including photocopying,
recording, or any information storage or retrieval system, without prior
permission in writing from the publishers.

Bloomsbury Publishing Plc does not have any control over, or responsibility for,
any third-party websites referred to or in this book. All internet addresses given
in this book were correct at the time of going to press. The author and publisher
regret any inconvenience caused if addresses have changed or sites have
ceased to exist, but can accept no responsibility for any such changes.

A catalogue record for this book is available from the British Library.

A catalog record for this book is available from the Library of Congress.

ISBN:	HB:	978-1-3503-4730-4
	ePDF:	978-1-3503-4732-8
	eBook:	978-1-3503-4731-1

Typeset by Integra Software Services Pvt. Ltd.

To find out more about our authors and books visit www.bloomsbury.com
and sign up for our newsletters.

For family and friends
along the via athletae

Contents

List of Figures	x
Preface	xi
Entitled and Embodied	xi
Running Order	xiv
Chapter Outline	xix
Foreword by Paul Allain	xxvii
Acknowledgements	xxxii
Note on Text	xxxiii
Introduction	1
We Are All Alligators	1
i. Bodyworld	2
Bodyworld and the 3As	2
Bodies in the Open	5
ii. Bodyworld Affordances in Sports	9
Affordances in Action	9
Intentionality in Affordance	12
iii. *Via Athletae* in Sports and Aesthetic Performance	14
Heart Athletes and Flying Acrobats	16
Action in Life	18
Action in the Boxing Ring	21
Punches in the Face of Ethics and Reality	24
Enduring Humanity	27
Part I Mind Games	
1 I Perform, I Think: Bodyworld Cognitions	33
Thinking About It	33
Mind Mapping	36
Attentional Focus	39
Movement Aesthetic and Economy	41
Outward Monitoring	44

viii   *Contents*

	Running Bodyworld	46
	Distraction	48
	Automatic Pilot and Exhaustion	51
	What I Take With Me	54
2	**Mind Your Body: Attentional Focus in Performance**	57
	Internal/External Focus and the Mind–Muscle Connection	58
	Flow Automaticity	61
	Epistemic Actions in Performance	65
	Secondary Tasks	68
	Focused Distraction	71
	Practice Insights	73
	Cross-Sectional Perspectives for Actors and Athletes	75
3	**Maintaining the Pace: Action Planning for Performance**	79
	Central Governor and Anticipatory Regulation	79
	Psychobiological Model	82
	Perception of Effort	85
	Pacing	87
	Aesthetic Pacing	90
	Dynamic Modulation	92
	Calibrating Inner Action	95
	Grafting Insights	97

Part II Heart Matters

4	**Feeling Performance: Affect, Sensation, Emotion**	101
	Affect Theory and Affective Science	102
	Experience Emotion Episode	105
	Eliciting Conditions	107
	'More Than Just an Actor Dressing'	109
	Expressive or Communicative Outcomes	111
	Stage Fright	113
	Action Readiness	115
	Improvisation and Real-World Play	117

	Contents	ix

5	Performing Feeling: Action, Intention, Transformation	121
	From Action Readiness to Actional Outcomes	122
	Thought-Action	125
	'A Cat With Which I have Contact', or Intentionality	128
	Emotion Modulation	131
	Changing Oneself	133

6	Putting on an Act: Performance Through Experience	137
	Cognitive Processing	138
	Enacting Action	141
	Aesthetic Experience	143
	Experience Case Studies	146
	Case Study 1 (Training): Plastiques	147
	Case Study 2 (Training Performance): *Tekhnē Sessions*	150
	Case Study 3 (Running): Long Runs	152
	Case Study Reflections: Aesthetics in Athletics	155
	Case Study 4 (Performance): *Id-Descartes* and *Martyr Red*	157
	Improvisational Conclusions	161

Conclusion: Along the *Via Athletae*	167
Setting the Scene	167
Practise What You Preach	170
The Sphere Exercise	171
Along the *Via Athletae*: List and Commentary	174

References	182
Index	195

Figures

1 Third Movement of *Tekhnē Sessions* by Icarus Performance
   Project (ActionBase Studio, Malta, 2004)   151
2 *Id-Descartes* by Groups for Human Encounter (ActionBase
   Studio, Malta, 2001)   158
3 *Martyr Red* by Icarus Performance Project (Valletta Campus
   Theatre, Malta, 2013)   159
4 *Martyr Red* by Icarus Performance Project (Jarman Building,
   University of Kent, UK, 2013)   159
5 *Martyr Red* by Icarus Performance Project (Valletta Campus
   Theatre, Malta, 2013)   159
6 First Movement of *Tekhnē Sessions* by Icarus Performance
   Project (ActionBase Studio, Malta, 2004)   165

Preface

Entitled and Embodied

Titles are always a good starting point. They encapsulate essential aspects of what follows, providing a first glimpse of the horizon of expectations that gradually expands as we learn more about the thing they name. They are first impressions that invite, attract, and sometimes even challenge the reader. *Performer Training for Actors and Athletes* is no different.

While echoing in part the title of my previous monograph *Performer Training Reconfigured: Post-Psychophysical Perspectives for the Twenty-first Century* (2019), this is a different book in scope, content, and range. Nevertheless, the two are kindred volumes because both interrogate what it means to prepare and train as a performer in the early twenty-first century. *Performer Training for Actors and Athletes* develops the argument by delving deeper in *and* broadening the field of interest. It does so by echoing the previous book's premise to rethink performer training in the light of early twenty-first-century perspectives, specifically with reference to the human–non-human dichotomy that the dominant psychophysical paradigm in performer studies left unchallenged. If the flag-bearing and wide-ranging impetus of the earlier book reflects visionary and manifesto aspirations, the focused explorations of the present volume suggest a nuanced inspection of some of the most fertile areas in the study of performer training.

Performer Training for Actors and Athletes unfolds its argument in three principal ways. First, it crystallizes and streamlines the core point of *Performer Training Reconfigured* by zeroing in on the concept of 'bodyworld'. In doing so it marks the intra-active processual relationality of the body–mind–environment phenomenological and sociomaterial composite that I ascribe to performers. Second, the book incorporates sports, specifically athletic activity and in particular long-distance running, in its understanding of 'performer' and 'performance'. The aim is to deploy insights from different somatic fields for a fuller appreciation of performing, mainly in the aesthetic and athletic spheres but also more widely. Third, the theoretical and scientific scaffolding in *Performer Training for Actors and Athletes* is complemented, reinforced, and to an evident degree also shaped, by practical considerations as informed by the author's experience in physical theatre and athletic performance.

The title of the book refers to no less than three kinds of practitioners: *performers*, *actors*, and *athletes*. As this formulation of 'practice' might

xii   *Preface*

imply, the discussion is not restricted to compartmentalized parameters of technique typically associated with 'actor training' or 'athletic training'. Rather, it is conducted in the broader terms of *performing* and *performance*, be it aesthetic, sport, or, for that matter, daily behaviour as understood in performance studies (Schechner 2013: 1). As a consequence of this inter- and cross-disciplinary approach, the word 'actor' is not limited to practices of 'acting' with associations of psychological realism like those linked with Konstantin Stanislavski, but stands for 'aesthetic performers' more generally, including those in physical, devised, dance, and other movement-based theatres. Similarly, 'athlete' serves as an umbrella for participants in sports that entail physical agility, strength, speed, and/or endurance; that is, it is not restricted to track and field contests established on the skills of running, jumping, and throwing, but includes others such as football, boxing, cycling, and tennis. Although a recurrent reference point for athletic practice in the book is endurance running, mainly because, as argued further down, it brings out in bolder relief elements that are inherent in human action, other sports are also discussed or exemplified. Notwithstanding these general markers about 'performers', 'actors', and 'athletes', particularities of practice are underlined whenever the case demands it.

Regarding the second word in the title, 'training', other possible alternatives are 'practice' and 'processes', both of which fit the territory covered in the book. However, both lack the specificity of 'training' when it comes to this volume's emphasis on preparation and formation. And yet, to capture the overlapping variety of all these terms – for a kind of three-dimensional rendering – 'training' is here understood in an expanded sense that also encapsulates 'practice' and 'process'. *Training as practice* highlights the physiological, technical, and material infra-/structures that constitute the phenomena examined in the book, as well as the socio-cultural specificities that give rise to and shape these activities. *Training as process* underscores the temporal spread and depth of these events to mark not so much the 'content' but the *developmental* and *durational dimension* of the psycho, physical, and affective qualities involved, i.e. the prior, during, and after of training.

The term 'reconfigured' in the title of my previous monograph referred to the radical interventions required to counter the human-centric approaches that characterize accounts of performer training. In the important endeavour to overcome mind–body dualisms, such narratives overlook human–non-human binaries, including those that pertain to human–environment, human–technology, and human–species, i.e. sets of reciprocally shaping *body–world* relationalities with their specific socio-cultural materialities. These human-centric accounts belong to a mind frame that needs updating to twenty-first-century imaginaries and realities. If I had to pick an equivalent

Preface xiii

word to accompany the present volume it would be 'reloaded'. While nodding at the aspirations of 'reconfigure' and its revisionary dynamics, *reloaded* shifts the emphasis from the constitutive 'rewiring' of the previous work to the positional 're-arrangement' and structural 'reinforcing' of these newly 'wired' elements. More pertinently, 'reloaded' connotes 'refreshing' and fine-tuning, specifically in the context of computing to fetch the latest updated version of a web page or document. If *reconfigure* plays on the 'figure' – and thus on the reconceptualization – of the human body, the internet overtones of *reload* evoke technology and its ubiquity, including in the perception, assessment, and prediction of performance, thus nuancing the intensified intra-existence of the 'performer training' body with the world in the twenty-first century (Kapsali 2021; Camilleri 2015a).

Although the term does not feature in the title, this is a book about 'bodyworld', for this concept is *illustrated by* as much as it *illustrates* my deliberations on performer training. As explained in the Introduction, its ever-present if subterranean currents inform the ensuing chapters. The compound word was first used in *Performer Training Reconfigured* to capture the body–mind–world fusion that constitutes the human agential intra-active relation with the world. In that book, bodyworld was expounded mainly in postphenomenological terms to analyse the impact of technology on human experience, but also in the light of situated cognition that conceives of knowing and knowledge as embodied and embedded as well as enacted or extended in the interaction between organism and material context. In the subsequent reception of the book, 'bodyworld' featured as a recurring point in personal feedback and critical reviews (e.g. Murphy 2019b; Spearman 2020: 186) – its concision and concretization touching a nerve especially in relation to the psychophysical 'bodymind' it updates. The interest in bodyworld led me to look closely at its composition and implications by situating it in specific instances of practice. Consequently, three articles appeared in 2020 to exemplify bodyworld in the context of mask work and the senses (Camilleri 2020a), puppetry and object performance (Camilleri [2020] 2022), and hybrid embodiment and gym machines (Camilleri 2020b). For present purposes, 'bodyworld' is often used in this book as a synonym for 'body' to foreground human–non-human constituent dimensionalities as well as to avoid body–world dualisms.

The perspectival emphasis in *Performer Training for Actors and Athletes* can also be traced to the diversity of viewpoints in every chapter of *Performer Training Reconfigured*. However, what distinguishes the two is the orientation of these outlooks: if the earlier book consists of 'post-psychophysical perspectives' borrowed from other disciplines to 'rewire' the study of performer training (e.g. postphenomenology, sociomateriality, work and organization studies, affect theory, and situated cognition), the present volume settles on 'bodyworld perspectives' as an *instance* of that 'rewiring', specifically as informed by athletic practice and sports science to emphasize, elaborate on, and exemplify the body in training and performance.

'Performer Training Reloaded: Bodyworld Perspectives for Actors and Athletes' was the original longer title that informed the research and first drafts of this book. However, as the writing of the chapters progressed, it became evident that although the implicit driving force of the argument remained 'bodyworld perspectives', the foregrounding of material processes necessitated by sports and athletic activity shifted the accent towards 'practices of doing' rather than their framing. These material processes included the physical and the physiological (i.e. the body and its functions), the mental and the psychological (i.e. the embodied mind and emotions), the technical and aesthetic (i.e. the matter and manner of training). However, one always perceives, thinks, and acts – and therefore *writes* – from a specific place. In the case of *Performer Training for Actor and Athletes*, that place is marked by the mutually shaping and signifying relations of bodyworld.

Running Order

Performer Training for Actor and Athletes is also written from a place of practice. I have been involved in theatre since 1989, specializing in research and training processes, always reflecting about and articulating my studio experience in diaries and performance programmes. Although I have operated in autonomous (non-institutional) contexts, I trace my influences to Jerzy Grotowski, Eugenio Barba, and Ingemar Lindh (Camilleri 2010: 161) via an apprenticeship and intense collaboration with John J. Schranz and projects with Lech Raczak in the 1990s. In 2001, I set up Icarus Performance Project (Malta), a group structure active under different guises and which follows an ongoing research laboratory that focuses on the space between training and performance processes (Icarus Performance Project 2022). Since 2004 I have found a base in academia that enables me to pursue a hybrid laboratory–scholarly practice. Icarus develops its practice research by means of two branches: devised performances and technical/experimental structures (Camilleri 2017). As the case studies in Chapter 6 demonstrate, both branches explore the interplay of training and performance via improvisation processes.

One of the analytical perspectives adopted in *Performer Training Reconfigured* comes from work and organization studies, which is deployed to shine a light on the 'invisible hours' that contribute to a holistic picture

Preface xv

of a 'work practice' (Camilleri 2019: 133, 2013a: 158–9). In the case of my theatre practice, these 'invisible hours' include the considerable time of reflection and writing about the studio activity, which is important 'work' in its own right because it filters experience and shapes subsequent training, rehearsals, and performances. Also 'invisible' is the 'non-theatre work' like martial arts and Latin American dance that I engaged in for different periods in my formation according to my technical and sometimes even devising/compositional needs. I considered these trainings as part of my theatre practice in developing the awareness and flexibility – and therefore the *psychophysical capacities* – of my embodiment. The most invisible of all, however, were the hours of running I had accumulated since I started my theatre journey in 1989.

As I have already published substantially about my theatre work (e.g. Camilleri and Schranz 1996; Camilleri 2004, 2010, 2013a, 2013c, 2013d, 2017, 2018b, 2019; Icarus Performance Project 2022), it is appropriate to elaborate on the 'athletic' aspect of my practice, which, recreational as it may be, has been consistently – if silently – pursued over more than three decades. The references to my practice in this book, including the case studies in Chapter 6, are not intended as a generalization or standard for either aesthetic or athletic practice. They are an additional resource that I, as author, cannot ignore, especially when writing about the cognitive and emotional dimensions of experience. As such, they are a disclosure of the bodyworlds that have informed the writing of this book. Another parameter or limitation concerns the fact that my running is autotelic (for the inherent sake of the activity) rather than competitively driven, which does not mean that I do not constantly challenge myself. Although this may be viewed as a crucial 'lack' in athletic practice, I have employed it methodologically as a defamiliarization strategy precisely to get to the fundamentally autotelic playfulness of sports. These and related issues are clarified and problematized in the course of the book.

I have often wondered why running was so invisible in the holistic conception of my theatre practice. Perhaps its 'athletic' (cardiovascular) activity rendered it too physiologically and mechanically functional compared to the 'aesthetic' forms of other non-theatre training I did (like taekwondo, tai chi, and salsa classes), somehow impairing its 'artistic' legitimacy. The repetitive act of putting one foot in front of another may have felt too basic and 'non-technical' to be of any relevance. Or maybe I considered it as 'me time', free from having to focus on 'learning a skill', allowing me to reset, daydream, gather my thoughts, or contemplate an issue that needed resolving as the endorphins started firing. In retrospect, and as is apparent in the following chapters, these are exactly some of the reasons why

xvi *Preface*

I find running appealing in my current research, i.e. *the essentialized quality of movement and the attendant cognitive activity that comes with running*. In other words, the full-body engagement that accompanies the continuous repetition of one step after another in accelerated time and extended space has the potential to illuminate fundamental dimensions of other psychosomatic practices that are more elaborate in their presentation. These dimensions, which revolve around the mobilization of the body as a whole, include intentionality, technique, and body–world relationality. Going out for a run is, indeed, an *essentialized* improvisation within a spatio-temporal structure, where one interacts with the world around and with oneself.

I can recognize a shift in the visibility of my running *as a practice* when I started using a mobile phone app in 2015 that tracked my performance in terms of distance covered, pace, elevation, etc. This enabled a different *perception* of running (Camilleri 2019: 76–8). However, my activity patterns remained more or less the same as before: circa two or three 6 km/30-minute runs a week, except for very occasional longer distances. The leap in perception and engagement came in late 2019, around six months after I acquired a Garmin sports watch and a chest heart rate monitor, when I started running ever longer distances and realized I could complete a half-marathon. I had long resisted running a competitive half-marathon because I thought I was 'old' and did not have the time or motivation to commit seriously to it. I *felt* that I could not run more than 6 km and needed at least two days to recover. Later I realized this was a fable I told myself and which I believed as truth – after all, I was the 'physical theatre' expert who had been 'working on oneself' for decades.

The deflation I felt when I finished the Malta Half-Marathon in March 2020, that I could have run longer and/or faster, did it for me: I immediately set myself the task of running a solo marathon, a standard I had previously thought unrealistic but which I managed to do two months later. This was when Covid made landfall in Europe, so swathes of time and space became available as we shifted to online work and the streets emptied. I invested time and effort in the activity, generously so with almost daily runs but also naively because I was not really following a plan except for some occasional suggestions from more experienced friends. That naïveté was in the main intentional because, influenced by my autodidacticism in theatre (Camilleri 2015a: 22–3), I resisted predetermined regimens so that I could explore this new territory in my own way before embarking on more structured and tested approaches. The risk of reinventing the wheel was worth taking because, as *personal invention*, I have found the learning process to be deeper and more lasting. Moreover, there is always something specific to – indeed, *of* – the individual when a wheel is (re)invented idiosyncratically. I learnt a

Preface xvii

great deal about myself, running, and the right equipment during this period, especially the value of preparation, pacing, and recovery, at times paying the price with bruised feet, broken toenails, aching muscles, dehydration, and niggling injuries.

For a statistical picture about my commitment as made available by the tracking apps, from a yearly average of running 850 km between 2015 and 2019, I increased to over 3000 km per annum in the 2020–2022 period. In terms of hours, this equates annually to 73 hours in 2015–2019 and 265 hours in 2020–2022 (excluding an average of three total recovery weeks after gruellingly long runs), thus approximating an increase from 1.5 hours to 5.5 hours every week just in running time. This difference has not only rendered visible what was previously invisible in my psychophysical practice, it also created a new category of 'running invisibility' for the hours of preparation (planning routes, mental readiness, and cross-training like walking, yoga, weights, and massages) and reflection (including note-taking and analysing the app data). Especially for my 50+ age group, I am an average runner as reflected in my best performance times of 19:31 minutes for 5 km, 1:38:13 for the half-marathon, and 3:24:26 for the marathon.

Early on in my recent engagement with the sport I had decided on running *longer* rather than *faster* as a more realistic challenge for my physiological and socio-cultural bodyworld. Having such an objective was one of the most important lessons I learnt at this stage because one always needs an ontology and a teleology, a becoming and a purpose, when embarking on a journey, even if the journey itself is the destination that dynamically adapts to one's progress. At the time of writing in early 2023, I have run ten solo and three competitive marathons (as well as countless 20+ km and 30+ km distances) in thirty months, always refining a personalized training programme that has now settled into four or five sessions a week (speed, steady, hill, easy, and long runs) plus additional slots for stretching, light weights, and, when possible, walks. During this period I have also run distances of 45 km, 50 km, and 52 km because the focus is always on pushing the endurance element. This has entailed changes to my training programme; for example, more recovery sessions now that 4-hour 42 km runs have become a 'training distance' rather than a 'performance distance', which makes a difference to the perception of effort, and hence to preparation and pacing strategy.

If I had to pick one aspect from my running activity that has altered the way I look at somatic practices, whether aesthetic or athletic, it will have to be, paradoxically, the mind. Ever since I began my theatre journey in 1989, I had been inculcated in the psychophysical belief that, as the inalienable medium of expression in aesthetic performance, the body is what primarily and ultimately matters, that the body is not subservient to the mind.

xviii   *Preface*

I accepted this perspective religiously because it was ubiquitous, thus even conditioning my own experience in the studio. However, in the rush and zeal to reject Cartesian dualism we tend to throw the proverbial baby out with the bath water, hence the foregrounding of the mind in Part I of this book, which was not planned but emerged as my research evolved in the streets and in the literature.

As 'Part I: Mind Games' makes amply clear, studies in sports science time and again point to the central role played by the mind in the body-field of athletic endeavour. My long-distance running has already taught me in no uncertain terms the crucial importance of the mind – not necessarily and exclusively of 'psychology' but of a mind with a nervous system that is as *physical* and *material* as the rest of the body. This has important implications, especially when it comes to intentionality and, paradoxically, automaticity in expert performance. The fable I had manufactured and believed that I could only run 6 km at a time, along with the walls I tore down with every milestone I covered (from 21 km to 24 km to 27 km to 30 km to 35 km to 37 km to 42 km to 45 km to 50 km to 52 km), are but manifestations of the mental dimension of embodiment. This has made me appreciate from a different angle the emphasis of theatre-maker Ingemar Lindh on mental precision in the physical act, especially when he distinguishes it from psychology, motivation, and related phenomena (see Chapter 5). In short, body and mind are indeed incontestably one, but aesthetic practices like theatre and dance stand to benefit from a reconsideration of the role played by the mind as crystallized in athletics and sports.

Running is aptly placed to analyse athletic endeavour and its implications, not only because it is 'a principal component of many other sports' (Bragaru et al. 2012: 294), but also because of its biomechanical dynamics and physiological qualities. Like standing up and walking, running arguably presents a 'pure' form of human activity in terms of its essentialized nature. Firstly, insofar as it involves the 'body only' (especially the barefoot or minimalist variety), it requires no additional technology or object, thus marking a fundamental relationship between body and world. Secondly, it is not only the body that is stripped of accoutrements but the activity itself: it consists of a simple and basic action that most humans can do in daily life. In this sense, running has primordial credentials, marking a fundamental characteristic of human embodiment. This makes it also relevant to aesthetic performance because, as an enabler of movement, it spotlights essential elements of action, behaviour, intentionality, affordance, and decision making – all elements that are tackled in *Performer Training for Actors and Athletes*.

Standing upright, with the specific positioning of the spine and bipedalism required by walking and running, is intimately associated with

Preface

being human. Biologist Dennis M. Bramble and paleoanthropologist Daniel E. Lieberman have investigated the performance of long-distance running and its evolution as an eminently human trait (Bramble and Lieberman 2004). Their comparative study of extinct hominins suggests that running played a key role in human evolution (Cregan-Reid 2016: 44). For example, in the words of Christopher McDougall when interviewing Lieberman:

> Our heads didn't just expand because we got better at running [...]; we got better at running because our heads were expanding, thereby providing more ballast. 'Your head works with your arms to keep you from twisting and swaying in midstride,' Dr. Lieberman said. The arms, meanwhile, also work as a counterbalance to keep the head aligned. 'That's how bipeds solved the problem of how to stabilize a head with a movable neck. It's yet another feature of human evolution that only makes sense in terms of running.'
>
> (McDougall 2010: 225)

It is only very recently in human evolution, in the last couple of centuries compared to the preceding 'millions of years', that we have become accustomed to mechanized transportation and even more lately to all sorts of cushioned footwear, including for running. Such changes, which reflect the wider innovations of industrialization and technologization, alienate us from the direct connection with the environment that has *adapted our bodies* to move, including to run, in certain ways. Bramble and Lieberman's research has revealed that, since evolution is 'tectonically slow', our bodies are still built for running and will take a *very* long time to adapt to these new circumstances (Cregan-Reid 2016: 43, 47).

Endurance of the kind epitomized by long-distance running appeals to my interest in the training of embodiment because, in pushing this body of ours to the limits of performance, it crystallizes and etches out in higher relief elements and aspects that are inherent (if concealed or less pronounced) in other practices, be they aesthetic, athletic, or quotidian, irrespective of body shape and condition. These dimensions of skilled embodiment include cognition and affect, the topics of Part I and Part II respectively, which brings me to the contents of this volume.

Chapter Outline

Performer Training for Actors and Athletes presents its case in two parts of three chapters each, framed by a conceptually and historically contextualizing introduction and a conclusion that compiles some of the practical implications of the aesthetic–athletic resonances in the volume. The trajectory of the book moves spirally forward, returning to certain motifs from different angles, thus developing and refining the focus on training from body to mind to emotion. From the general, focused, and strategic cognitions of Part I, to the sensori-emotionally emergent, actional, and modulating behaviour of Part II, the volume paints a multi-dimensional picture of the performing body-in-the-world.

The Introduction prepares the ground in three main segments, starting with a conceptualization of the body–world relationalities that constitute human experience, moving on to an appraisal of these dimensions as action possibilities in sports, and concluding on a comparative analysis with theatre practice that leads to a consideration of broader implications for athletic and aesthetic processes. The first section, 'Bodyworld', refers to the performer's entangled engagement with the material world in terms of assemblages, their affordances, and socio-cultural status. This is exemplified by a focus on outdoor practices to highlight the material and ecological basis of human activity that is often overlooked in indoor settings. The second section, 'Bodyworld Affordances in Sports', develops the argument with an overview from embodied cognition of the coupling of athletes with real-world scenarios. Connections between perception and action, as well as intentionality and decision making, are evoked within the frame of skilled behaviour. The third section, '*Via Athletae* in Sports and Aesthetic Performance', deals with dimensions in aesthetic practice that can be aligned with skilled athletic endeavour. The discussion unfolds within a historical contextualization prompted by Antonin Artaud's notion of an actor's 'affective athleticism' and Franco Ruffini's analysis of theatre and boxing. Implications for practice, including overlaps with competitiveness and play, are explored by the proposal of a 'way of the athlete' where corporeal truth to material reality in aesthetic, athletic, and daily practices is directly linked to bodyworld affordances and ethical sensibility.

'Part I: Mind Games' examines the 'mind' aspect of the bodyworld assemblages in athletic and aesthetic performance. This emphasis is in part due to the endeavour in theatre and dance studies to shift the focus of analysis in performer process on to the somatic with the result that the mental dimension is often overlooked, no doubt to compensate for the privileged position it has historically occupied in the Cartesian West and that still conditions conceptions of the body. However, a fresh approach to the roles played by the mind, especially as provided by sports science in the context of the explicit physicality of athletic practice, lights the matter in different hues. Apart from marking the mind/body connection, the chapter titles in Part I trace the overall progression of argument: from Chapter 1's

Preface xxi

appraisal of generalized 'cognitions' or 'thoughts' during movement, to Chapter 2's mobilization of 'attentional focus', to Chapter 3's more structured and strategic metacognitive processes of 'action planning'.

Chapter 1, 'I Perform, I Think: Bodyworld Cognitions', focuses on the bodyworld of actors and athletes from the perspective of cognition, specifically as prompted by the kind of mental activities that occur during running. The chapter seeks to capture the specificities of the various types of cognitive phenomena typically investigated by sports science, here as categorized by sports exercise psychologist Noel Brick, including internal sensory monitoring, active self-regulation, outward and environmental monitoring, as well as active and involuntary distraction. This insight is juxtaposed with conceptualizations of awareness from aesthetic performer practice, mainly Phillip Zarrilli's embodied modes of experience, but also as featured in the work of Thomas Richards, Roberta Carreri, and the author. The cross-lighting of athletic and aesthetic processes is aimed at a more concrete understanding of the cognitions that characterize the performing body, principally concerning connections and differences between movement aesthetic and movement economy as well as with regard to automaticity and exhaustion. The quality of movement in terms of economy/efficiency and automaticity/modality are recurrent themes in the book that are first tackled in this chapter.

Chapter 2, 'Mind Your Body: Attentional Focus in Performance', continues the re-evaluation of the embodied mind in somatic practices. It specifically explores matters relating to attentional focus, the 'mind–muscle connection', and behavioural automaticity. The argument is framed by Gabriele Wulf's distinction from sports science between external and internal references in attentional focus, which builds on Chapter 1's mapping of cognitive activities. The 'mind–muscle connection' in resistance training is juxtaposed with psychophysicality in aesthetic processes with the aim of illuminating the question of inner and outer actions from a different angle. The point is further examined via behavioural automaticity, specifically with reference to 'choke' and flow experiences. While an internal focus is viewed as triggering typical 'choking' episodes through self-evaluative and self-regulatory processing, the switch to a paradoxically unconscious mode of control in expert performers is considered from the point of Mihaly Csikszentmihalyi's optimal flow experience. In this regard, the roles of 'epistemic' (or indirect) actions in aesthetic performance and 'secondary tasks' in sports are discussed in the context of a more nuanced appraisal of intentional distraction that is sometimes engaged to enhance athletes' performance, in the process providing a different take on automaticity in aesthetic performance.

Chapter 3, 'Maintaining the Pace: Action Planning for Performance', develops the discussion about the mind/body relationalities in athletic and

xxii   *Preface*

aesthetic world-contexts. It examines in more depth the paradoxical interplay identified in the preceding chapter between attention and automaticity in performance. Accordingly, psychological and physiological aspects related to conscious and non-conscious dimensions are explored with regard to two major outlooks in sports science: Tim Noakes's central governor theory and Samuele Marcora's psychobiological model of perceived effort. The argument is illustrated with reference to pacing in endurance sports and to its adaptation for aesthetic processes. 'Aesthetic pacing' is proposed within the frame of organizational structures in theatre and dance performances, mainly as prompted by Eugenio Barba's understanding of the multi-levels of performance scores, all of which require the organization-in-motion of 'pacing' when presented to an audience. The conceptualization of 'aesthetic pacing' highlights the potential benefits of deploying insights from athletics and sports science to aesthetic performance, and vice versa. Within this chapter, pacing is considered as a sophisticated instance of *planning by* and *of action* – and it is this preparatory 'planning' and its ongoing 'regulation' during the event that highlights aspects of cognition and attentional focus in Part I.

Following Part I's emphasis on the mental dimension in athletic and aesthetic practices, 'Part II: Heart Matters' focuses on *feeling* and its attendant sensorial and emotional qualities that condition perception and action. As a continuously emergent phenomenon in the relational exchange between bodies and world, affect is identified in the optimally placed liminal space between inside and outside. The appraisal of affect is based on a reading of affect theory as informed by affective science, i.e. two outlooks that are rarely considered in the light of each other due to terminological, analytical, and application divergences but which together provide a fuller picture of felt perception and its implications for aesthetic, sport, and daily performance. Accordingly, Patrick Colm Hogan's reading from affective science of the various stages in an *emotion episode* are adopted as an itinerary across the three chapters in Part II, with Chapter 4 tackling *eliciting conditions*, *expressive outcomes*, and *action readiness*; Chapter 5 covering *actional outcomes* and *emotion modulation*; and Chapter 6 concluding on *cognitive processing* and *phenomenological tone*. The rationalization of emotion as an episodic development of sensorial perception and interpretation offers a productive analytical viewpoint on psychophysical practices.

Chapter 4, 'Feeling Performance: Affect, Sensation, Emotion', begins with an understanding of feeling in terms of preconscious affect, sensory sensation, and processed emotion as they feature and overlap in emotion episodes. To illustrate a case of *eliciting conditions* in the bodyworld of performers, the use of equipment is considered. From footwear for runners

Preface xxiii

to costumes in Stanislavski, equipment highlights the material relationality in existing conditions and in potential variables in all practices, including as it intersects with the concept of 'enclothed cognition'. The second component in an emotion episode, *expressive or communicative outcomes*, consists of unplanned somatic reactions that convey a feeling or an emotion to others. The uncontrollable experience of 'stage fright' in aesthetic performance, which parallels 'choking' in athletic practice, provides some insight into a specific set of communicative outcomes. The next stage, *action readiness*, deals with a form of physiological 'priming' that prepares the performing body for action (e.g. the tensing of relevant muscles for a specific action). Action readiness is discussed via the dynamics of play and games, in particular with reference to improvisation in aesthetic performance (specifically, Jacques Lecoq's *le jeu*) and real-world practice in sports.

Chapter 5, 'Performing Feeling: Action, Intention, Transformation', focuses on *actional outcomes* as the mid-way component in the categorization of emotion episodes. As the feature that spectators see on stage and in sports, actional outcomes are important, also because they manifest the processes that precede them in an episode and serve as the operating material for the ones that follow. Distinguishing between *action readiness* and *actional outcomes*, reference is made to isometry, a type of sports exercise where no movement is visible despite muscular activation. Ingemar Lindh's adaptation of isometry in his theatre research on intentionality is considered in the light of Étienne Decroux's 'mobile immobility', especially as it overlaps with what Eugenio Barba denotes by the integrated thought-action of *sats* (impulses and counter-impulses). Jerzy Grotowski's understanding of 'body memory' is evoked in the context of emotionally charged phenomena like memories and associations that accompany the muscular activation and mental mobilization of intention. An example of *emotion modulation* as the regulation of emotional response is discussed with reference to a sports science study on the impact of facial expressions on movement economy and perceptual responses during running. Some implications for aesthetic performance are explored.

Chapter 6, 'Putting on an Act: Performance Through Experience', brings the discussion on emotion episodes to a close with the two remaining aspects of actional outcomes. Due to their reciprocal conditioning, *cognitive processing* and *phenomenological tone* are considered together in the light of each other. An additional aim of the chapter is to draw on various insights from Parts I and II for a holistic picture of the aspects examined in the book. Following an exposition on cognitive processing and embodiment, which includes Maiya Murphy's enactivist assessment of Jacques Lecoq's pedagogy in aesthetic performance, the chapter proceeds to phenomenological tone xxiv *Preface*

by means of four case studies from the author's aesthetic and athletic practices. Dealing with a training exercise, a hybrid training/performance structure, long runs, and two physical theatre scenes, the case studies focus on a specific phenomenological tonality in the aesthetic and athletic space of improvisation with deeply assimilated material. Aesthetic elements in athletic behaviour are highlighted via the awareness/cognition and modulation/regulation of one's 'form', understood as the felt perception of one's psychophysical condition. Distinct from the 'interpretation' (however masterful) of existing scores and techniques, the *compositional* implications of 'creative' solutions foregrounded by automaticity in improvisation are also discussed as liberatory, including as they overlap with Mihaly Csikszentmihalyi's optimal 'flow' experiences.

The Conclusion, 'Along the *Via Athletae*', revisits the Introduction's proposal of a modality of performing that is not based on a specific technique or method but on the intensity of psychophysical commitment. This *via athletae* engagement is manifested in the dynamics of (1) *play* as autotelic activity, (2) collaborative *competitiveness* in its etymological sense of 'flying with', and (3) *pacing* as an organizational and management framework during performance. The chapter begins with a deconstruction of assumptions regarding the 'reality' and 'truth' of skilled action for a nuanced understanding of certain modalities of trained behaviour, which in turn sheds light on aesthetic, athletic, and daily practices more generally. By compiling key aspects from the preceding chapters that align with *via athletae*, the rest of the Conclusion considers some implications for practice. To this end, the author's Sphere Exercise, which works on awareness within a physical and imaginative context that improves intentionality, illuminates the 'Along the *Via Athletae*' list that follows it. The emphasis on structures and dynamics underlines the 'inhabited' or 'worked upon' dimension associated with *via athletae* as a modality of skilled doing that is the rule not the exception in human behaviour.

*

A reviewer of an early version of the above chapter outline drew attention to two aspects that shed further light on the character of this volume: (1) the 'individuality of optimization' vis-à-vis different bodies and (2) the role of the voice.

In more ways than one, including as it overlaps with my other publications, the book's focus on the awakening of the optimal body in performance indeed concerns the 'individuality of optimization' in performer training, regardless of the normative, ideal, 'fit' body that is generally associated with

Preface xxv

athleticism and elite sports. The Introduction opens with a discussion on dis/ability via the example of an anthropomorphized alligator whose body does not 'fit in' in a human world, thus the section heading 'We Are All Alligators'. The alligator is a metaphor for the kind of human body that is understood by and addressed in the book. This is a body that, as I argue and take my cue from Karen Barad, is always in a prosthetic relationship with the world due to the organization of and dependence on the inhabited environment. Hence the emphasis on the concepts of bodyworld and affordances. As such, this opening discussion sets the tone for the rest of the book's consideration of bodies and their optimization.

Furthermore, my proposal of *via athletae* addresses in direct and specific ways the 'individuality of optimization' in performer training. It does so via the selection and actualization of the *affordances* of one's body, irrespective of its form and qualities, whether fat or thin, disabled or even chronically ill. This is particularly evident in the practical treatment of *via athletae* in the Conclusion, where I elaborate on an exercise that does not presuppose but aspires towards technical proficiency according to one's body and abilities. In this regard, the featured exercise in the Conclusion complements Case Study 1 (Chapter 6) that deals with a training accessible to various bodies in being based on certain principles that can be embodied differently. The question this volume foregrounds is not so much the accessibility and inclusivity of training but its *proficiency* according to the potential capacity and actualized ability – the *affordances* – of one's body.

Although the role of the voice may not be explicit at first glance, it is certainly present as a perusal of the relevant index entries demonstrates. The holistic perspective encouraged in the book strongly implies and includes the voice when talking about the actor's body and experience. For example, Case Study 4 (Chapter 6) deals with a song in my solo performance *Id-Descartes*. See also the various references to stage fright, which concern exclusively the use of the voice on stage. Then there is the dimension of 'Expressive or Communicative Outcomes' (Chapter 4) that involves involuntary vocalizations which may still be deployed consciously and strategically in certain instances in aesthetic, athletic, and daily behaviour. In all these scenarios, the voice is integrated with the physical and emotional body of the performer.

The issue of the voice's visibility (or rather 'audibility') is related to a matter of focus and remit. Most probably, it reflects the nature of the voice's minimal deployment in sports, which does not mean that it has no role to play. For example, the Introduction considers Brendan Ingle's idiosyncratic training for championship-winning boxers that included singing during punching routines. In one sense, athletes are like traditional dancers and mimes who perform without engaging the voice in public performances. It is no coincidence that the book makes substantive references to mime practitioners like Étienne Decroux and Jacques Lecoq, both of whom were influenced by Jacques Copeau who, as we also see in the Introduction, focused on corporeal improvisation in his innovative training for actors that also involved the voice.

Foreword

If I were to compare this book to a sport, and more specifically a competitive run perhaps, I am uncertain which it would be. It's definitely not a 100-metre dash. Nor does it feel like a marathon, and certainly not an ultramarathon, an extraordinary phenomenon to which this text introduced me. It's not a jog, at least from my chair-bound perspective as I write this. It's probably more akin to a systematic, well-prepared for, focused 20 km run that takes the runner (in this instance the reader) to a surprising new location. This endpoint is also a beginning, a world of reflection home to insights carefully gathered from sports science that are deployed to enrich physical actor training, historically the more familiar terrain of Frank Camilleri's research.

If I had to decide what kind of performance *Performer Training for Actors and Athletes* might be, I would struggle even more. Camilleri carefully points out how, moving on from physicality in common, the domain of creative expressivity in training for actors has scant relation to the strictures of sports, with their teleological imperatives, narrow parameters, and scientific measures. Performance does not operate according to objective scientific conditions, as theatre and performance researchers know only too well. And although both share several terms such as 'training' and 'performing', this creative imperative is mostly where they depart. This is less true of forms such as gymnastic dance, an 'aesthetic' as opposed to 'purposive' sport, but it is nevertheless still a useful general distinction.

Camilleri probes both differences and similarities between acting and athletics with a forensic sensibility. The interface between these two areas is largely what the book explores: that point where physical activity stops being about oxygen levels, lactic acid build-up, or muscular stress and moves into a creative and imaginative realm. The mind is inevitably deeply involved in athletics and its training and cannot be ignored. But, Camilleri argues, in much theatre and sports research alike in recent years, the somatic aspect has been foregrounded perhaps to the detriment of fully understanding mental processes. Camilleri sets out to change this.

Differences aside, ways of preparing for a sporting event share much with those for the performing arts. For me, this connection emerged first through the practice of night running in which I participated in the early 1990s with Gardzienice Theatre Association in the small Polish village of this name, encompassing an activity which is central to this book. Night running was conducted in a group along the village's sandy pine forest paths as dusk

xxviii *Foreword*

fell. It was conducted at a slow pace, supported by articulated rhythmical breathing, interspersed with pauses for singing, sounding, or other exercises such as group or pair acrobatics. For Gardzienice, night running is not only part of but also leads into further training and rehearsal. It acts as a liminoid segue from daily chores and working life into the night-time process (for this group at least) of creative exploration, the outcomes of which, their performances, have been acclaimed internationally. Night running shifts into and incarnates the optimal flow that allows altered and heightened perceptions and physicalities, so vital for the creative process. Gardzienice's practice has been hugely influential and significant worldwide, even if serious misconduct accusations against the director have recently cast a pall over this. Regrettably, sports and performing arts share this in common too.

Thanks to this book, I now understand much more about what was going on when I was running in Poland. Today when I pick up a racket to play social tennis outdoors in a Kentish village, I reflect more: not during the game, for that would lead to self-consciousness and possible 'choking', which Camilleri discusses in detail here. Rather, I reflect afterwards. Choking's closest equivalent in the performing arts is the more familiar idea of stage fright, which has attracted much attention recently in theatre scholarship. Fascinatingly, Camilleri positions these behaviours in parallel. I have never faced the paralysing effects of stage fright at my tennis club, but I am very aware of the stifling nervousness that can inhibit and take over when I go from a friendly club knockabout to a local league game with a rival village. I expect to win my next competitive game, theoretically armed and bodily aware as I now am!

There are many such rich affinities and congruences in this book. Camilleri offers numerous insights into techniques or terms deployed in high-level sports training and explores how these relate to acting. We have probably all wanted to be more focused on a set task at times or encouraged our students to be so. Focus is vital for the actor, but it is one of those words like 'energy' and 'presence' that is often quite intangible or hard to negotiate in practice. As teachers/trainers, we know that asking for more focus does not make it happen in a causal way. Camilleri examines usefully how notions like automaticity and distraction can both aid and hinder, and how such ideas interweave in this all-encompassing term. He artfully makes the complex clear. There are so many terms deployed here that are new to or recast for our field (phenomenological tone, actional outcomes, action readiness, emotion episode, perception of effort, attentional focus, and distraction to name but a few). It is best left for the book rather than this brief foreword to explain these, but, reader, be prepared to go back to things! A 20 km run does not happen without repetition, preparation, or practice.

Foreword xxix

As well as drawing extensively from sports research, Camilleri is as comfortable negotiating numerous theatrical reference points. These include Ingemar Lindh, Jerzy Grotowski, Eugenio Barba, Étienne Decroux, Jacques Copeau, and Jacques Lecoq. The last began his career in physical education, so is an understandable player in this book. Yet all of them have devoted their working lives to processes of actor training, emphasizing the physical. Readers familiar with Camilleri's writing will have heard much on and from these figures before. Here, though, they are brought into sharp and surprising relief through this new analytical frame of the athletic.

An emphasis on what we do, across both athletics and acting, grounds the book, and ample evidence from practice is offered to elucidate the range of terms and notions. As it moves through sometimes difficult theories and terminology, an authoritative voice emerges, shaped through learning gained from lived experience, from systematic doing. Camilleri has been obsessively running, evaluating, and reflecting, building on his equally systematic earlier decades as a theatre performer and in teaching and training, much of the latter being autodidactic. Whilst he has clearly thought a great deal and thought hard, he has recently been assisted by smart watches and the multiple means to which we can now all reach out in order to gain data on our very heartbeats, in the blink of an eye. Moving on again from the objective and scientific, the book ends with illuminating case studies from his own performances, yet it is also peppered throughout with observations drawn from life.

As well as such data-gathering and reflection, there are many other affordances that are analysed along the way, from specific high-tech athletic clothing and shoes to character costume, as well as the outdoor environment, its significance arising from the fact that running frequently happens in highly variable conditions outside. What better practice for improvisation and heightening awareness does one need than a jog through urban terrain. Covid has made us acutely sensitized to where things happen: for all its destruction, it has revitalized our engagement with the environment and fresh air, something this book also reinforces.

Camilleri is not afraid of facing into and tackling the harder questions, problems of feelings, emotions, perception, cognition. Perhaps we should not be surprised, given his writing in the book about regular runs of over 40 km, including several ones at 3 a.m. His wide reading in sports science yields a fertile interdisciplinarity. This book is no improvisation, and its findings arise from experiment, practice, and fundamentally hard work, in reading, interpreting, and analysing as much as running and acting.

Another strength is how the book relates to and builds on the author's overall body of work. Sceptics might initially baulk at the self-citation that

xxx *Foreword*

occurs throughout. But this is no vanity or introspection. Rather it is a considered and detailed attempt to extend and deepen ideas and arguments previously touched upon in several articles and books. He elaborates on his pioneering earlier use of the hybrid term 'bodyworld' which moved us on from Phillip Zarrilli's narrower bodymind, and also his detailed exegesis on 'habitation' as a mode of action. This idea of a body of work is particularly apposite in this context. The book splits into two sections, 'Mind Games' and 'Heart Matters' respectively, but it might be imagined as the prosthetic bionic limbs that reach out from and extend his previous work, including the very recent *Performer Training Reconfigured* (2019). This body also reveals Camilleri's extraordinary productivity, an academic ultramarathon par excellence!

Life often introduces surprising serendipities. I write this foreword whilst supporting an ambitious Greek project to establish performing arts, focused on acting, in the small town and district of Marathon outside Athens (Selioni 2022). Its aim is to develop an MFA in Acting that works across film and theatre, as well as summer festivals, schools, and research-related activities, all of which somehow respond to the world-renowned site. Marathon as a place never needs explaining, its role as the starting point for a 26.2 mile /42.195 km run firmly etched in history, location of the famous battle of the Greeks against the Persians from which this run derives. For the 2004 Athens Olympics, Marathon built extensive new facilities: a running track, gymnasium, reception areas, and a press office, and a vast concrete starting point for the world-famous race, overlooked by steps that lead up to a holder for the Olympic flame. This track accommodates the tens of thousands of runners who gather in November annually to repeat the race. Nearby is the Marathon Museum which houses running shoes, Olympic flame torches, and other archival material from Olympics from around the world and across decades.

This book looks way back in bringing sport and performance together again but also anticipates this new Greek aspiration. Camilleri does not write a cultural history of such connections across time, though he does touch briefly in the introduction on the Athenian Dionysia. Rather he focuses specifically on understanding what lessons we might learn from sports that can tell us something more about what acting is and what training can be. One key topic is pacing, a term which we might easily recognize as being central to both contexts. Pacing here is more than a dramaturgical structural dimension and is as much about intuiting and feeling, yet in a highly organized way. We train and practise in order to better know when and how pacing should or could change. Camilleri takes us deeply into explaining

Foreword

xxxi

what the processes are that allow us to know when to go faster, when to ease off, when to sustain, in theatrical performance as much as in sport.

The book concludes by bringing together 'Mind Games' and 'Heart Matters' in what Camilleri calls *via athletae*, a nod to Polish theatre director Jerzy Grotowski's *via negativa* with all its connotations of removing the actor's psychophysical blocks. Camilleri's 'way' is as much about becoming more precisely aware and thus better performers as it is about enhancing our sense of ourselves and how we interact with the world which shapes us – just as we shape it. Ultramarathons are at one extreme of this, as are durational or highly technical aesthetic performances like circus. Yet Camilleri writes for everyone, careful to eschew notions of elitism, emphasizing rather that we are only what we are, even if this might be altered through training, and that there are no ideal paradigms. This book examines how we all live, of which performing is one small part.

As I write, I cannot dispel from my mind the image and felt sense of that huge historic starting point in Marathon, a space that is functionally designed for thousands to run from but also framed and structured for viewing as much as doing. The mental image I hold somehow transports me back, almost physically. In my bodyworld, my mind travels and I am there in an instant. Camilleri's book is a thoughtful guide to all such travels, in body and mind.

Paul Allain
Canterbury, January 2023

Acknowledgements

This book would not have been possible without a number of presences in my life, including the ones below.

My parents, Luigia and Charles, and my brothers, Brian, Neville, and Christopher, for being there and shaping me.

My colleagues and friends in the Department of Theatre Studies, School of Performing Arts, at the University of Malta: Mario Frendo, Stefan Aquilina, Vicki Ann Cremona, and Marco Galea, for the shared experiences over the years.

Paul Allain, for the guidance, support, and companionship from 'Day 1'.

Nicole Bugeja, Felipe Cervera, Nesreen Hussein, and Judita Vivas, as well as Clive Ferrante and Elton Baldacchino, for 'running' with me in different ways.

Jeremy de Maria and Sandro Spina, for the 'insider' photography.

Carmel Serracino, for helping me with the Latin subtleties of '*via athletae*'.

Anna Brewer and Aanchal Vij at Bloomsbury, for steering me through the publication process, and the anonymous reviewers, for the constructive feedback.

Colleagues and students, past and present, for the opportunities to learn.

The Director of Finance and the Academic Resources Funds Committee at the University of Malta, for approving my request to use a substantial amount of my yearly allocation of research funds to the purchasing of running footwear.

Icarus Performance Project (Malta), for facing the sun.

Note on Text

This is not a book about actors. It is a book about actors *and* athletes.

Although I refer to various theoretical and scientific sources, I have tried to write accessibly for a broad readership. The lack of endnotes reflects the endeavour to make the text as self-explanatory as possible. In the same spirit, and mindful that readers from the performing arts and sports may not be aware of developments in each other's fields, I briefly introduce all cited authors and practitioners as well as contextualize all theories and concepts.

The several references to my other publications reflect the organic development of the connections and embodied/thought processes that have informed this book.

The 'Bodyworlds and the 3As' sub-section in the Introduction compiles and extends some of the relevant material about the subject from my previous writings. This material is reprinted by permission of the publisher (Taylor & Francis Ltd, http://www.tandfonline.com): Frank Camilleri, 'From Bodymind to Bodyworld: The Case of Mask Work as a Training for the Senses', *Theatre, Dance and Performance Training*, 11: 1 (2020); 'Of Assemblages, Affordances, and Actants – Or the Performer as Bodyworld: The Case of Puppet and Material Performance', *Studies in Theatre and Performance*, 42: 2 ([2020] 2022); 'A Hybridity Continuum: The Case of the Performer's Bodyworlds', *Performance Research*, 25: 4 (2020).

Material in Chapter 1 from Noel Brick, Tadhg MacIntyre, and Mark Campbell, 'Attentional Focus in Endurance Activity: New Paradigms and Future Directions', *International Review of Sport and Exercise Psychology*, 7: 1 (2014), is reprinted by permission of the publisher (Taylor & Francis Ltd, http://www.tandfonline.com).

Material in Chapter 2 from Gabriele Wulf, 'Attentional Focus and Motor Learning: A Review of 15 Years', *International Review of Sport and Exercise Psychology*, 6:1 (2013), is reprinted by permission of the publisher (Taylor & Francis Ltd, http://www.tandfonline.com).

Some paragraphs concerning Gunnar Borg's RPE Scale in Chapter 3 and on Affect Theory and Affective Science in Chapter 4 are adapted from my article 'Seeing it Feelingly: On Affect and Bodyworld in Performance', *New Theatre Quarterly*, 39: 1 (2023). This material has been modified to accommodate the context of the present publication. The application of this theoretical material is original to *Performer Training for Actors and Athletes*.

xxxiv *Note on Text*

Material in Chapter 5 from Frank Camilleri, "'To Push the Actor-Training to Its Extreme": Training Process in Ingemar Lindh's Practice of Collective Improvisation', *Contemporary Theatre Review*, 18: 4 (2008), is reprinted by permission of the publisher (Taylor & Francis Ltd, http://www.tandfonline.com).

Original spelling, punctuation, and reference conventions are retained in all cited material.

Introduction

We Are All Alligators

The work of Japanese artist Keigo offers defamiliarized perspectives of being in the world. His Instagram page, under the name of 'k5fuwa', is full of drawings and cartoon clips that, despite their naïve style, provide insight about *living* on earth. A case in point are his illustrations about the daily struggles of an anthropomorphized alligator trying to perform – and therefore to *fit* – in a human world, whether it is in sports, aesthetic performance, or daily life. From serving a tennis ball or hooping a basketball, to playing a violin or crashing cymbals, to climbing a ladder or having a CT scan, his snout keeps getting in the way of 'normal' human behaviour. Like the alligator's story, this book is about the embodied processes that athletes, actors, dancers, and other performers pursue in a material world.

The travails of Keigo's alligator foreground the point that the world we inhabit is formed, organized, or adapted according to the requirements of the human body, more precisely, to specific configurations that *enable* – and therefore privilege – that embodiment. This is evidenced by the roles we play in life, including not only quotidian and skilled behaviour but also the tools, technology, and infrastructure we develop to facilitate that corporeality, that *body-reality*. In such a world, alligators are 'dis-abled'. As feminist and physics theorist Karen Barad argues:

> The luxury of taking for granted the nature of the body as it negotiates a world constructed specifically with an image of "normal" embodiment in mind is enabled by the privileges of ableism. It is when the body doesn't work [or fit that it] then becomes clear that "able-bodiedness" is not a natural state of being but a specific form of embodiment that is co-constituted through the boundary-making practices that distinguish "able-bodied" from "disabled."
>
> (Barad 2007: 158)

In a parallel world designed for an other form of body, the 'normal' human body is 'disabled'. Barad claims that, being able-bodied in a world organized for able-bodies 'means being in a *prosthetic relationship* with the "disabled"', precisely because the environment props up that kind of being-body at various levels of existence (Barad 2007: 158, emphasis added). As the state of being-body, therefore, embodiment necessarily involves a body's material and 'prosthetic' relationship with the world.

Keigo's illustrations and Barad's reflections tell us that, as bodied entities, we are all alligators, i.e. beings with specific *material* (physical) bodies that inhabit specific *material* (environmental) contexts. *Such body–world interactions condition not only our socio-cultural who-we-are but also, symbiotically, the way we move, feel, think, and therefore our psychophysical embodiment.* In *Performer Training Reconfigured* (2019), I propose the '*post-psychophysical*' as an acknowledgement of the co-forming relationalities between bodies and the world. These reciprocally shaping connections are frequently, and systematically, overlooked in the psychophysical emphasis on body/mind integrity, aimed at overcoming that particular aspect of Cartesian dualism. Accordingly, the *post-psychophysical* promotes a critical awareness of psychophysicality as a perspective that gives rise to certain *forms of embodiment* at the expense of others. As such, the post-psychophysical recognition that the material context is not simply a 'background' but an *active and formative force* in the performer's work, has far-reaching implications. The present volume sheds light on this aspect of being human, irrespective of one's body, by focusing on what aesthetic and athletic performers foreground in their practices.

i. Bodyworld

Bodyworld and the 3As

At the heart of the post-psychophysical project is the concept of 'bodyworld', which refers to the performer's entangled engagement with the material world. 'Bodyworld' seeks to capture what eludes the psychophysical term 'bodymind' that, in aspiring to transcend the mind–body binary, leaves the human–non-human dichotomy unchallenged. First introduced in *Performer Training Reconfigured* (Camilleri 2019), the concept was subsequently developed and exemplified in other publications (Camilleri 2020a, 2020b, [2020] 2022). This section compiles and extends some of the relevant material from these sources.

As acknowledged in the Preface, 'bodyworld' is the implicit perspective adopted in this book. And it is a defamiliarizing term. We recognize the two elements that constitute the compound word but their fusion throws off balance our expectations of what 'body' and 'world' mean. In this text, 'bodyworld' is used as a synonym for 'body'. But what body or kind of body is it? Precisely, a 'body-in-the-world' that is pertinently *of* the world in being conditioned and constituted by it. Despite the apparent redundancy of this statement, we frequently conceive of bodies as if they are free-standing entities separate from the world around. As Keigo's illustrations demonstrate, we do not immediately and always see the 'in/of-the-world' qualities and dimensions of bodies due to the prosthetic infrastructure that props us up. To this end, the neologism 'bodyworld' foregrounds the reciprocally shaping connections between bodies and the worlds they inhabit, in the process also signalling the human–non-human relationalities that constitute experience.

The term fuses Phillip Zarrilli's psychophysical *bodymind* from the field of acting (Zarrilli 2009: 4) with Don Ihde's Husserl-inspired *lifeworld* from a postphenomenology that focuses on the impact of specific technologies on experience (Ihde 1990). Admittedly, the notion of 'bodyworld' resonates with those performance and somatic practices that examine the interrelation between body and environment. Such practices include paratheatre, Body Weather, and the interdisciplinary area of ecosomatics that, similar to Anna Halprin's work, connects embodiment disciplines like dance and healing arts with ecological consciousness. However, my proposal goes beyond the natural environment to include our lived urban, industrial, and technological conditions (Camilleri 2019: 35–43). Accordingly, the *world* in 'bodyworld' refers as much to the post-natural as to the natural world (Camilleri 2019: 63, Camilleri 2020a: 26).

Such an understanding of 'bodyworld' can be aligned, in part, with turn-of-the-twentieth-century German biologist Jakob von Uexküll's notion of *Umwelt* (literally, 'world around'), which denotes the environment *as perceived and acted upon* by living organisms, including the human animal. Uexküll distinguished *Umwelt* from *Umgebung*, the latter signalling the actual physiochemical surroundings of the organism. The *Umwelt* connection between sense-making *perception of* and *action in* the world – and therefore how the environment affects human behaviour and vice versa – captures an important dimension of bodyworld. It also anticipates Martin Heidegger's 'being-in-the-world' and enactive cognition's 'bringing forth of the world', both of which underscore in their different ways the inseparable connections between subject/object and inside/outside (Colombetti 2017: 447). Post-psychophysicality appreciates this inside/outside relationality not only as the integration of mind and body but, crucially, of mind/body *and world*.

In this regard it is worth quoting what postmodern artist, dancer, and choreographer Simone Forti (b. 1935) prefers to call 'body-mind-world' instead of 'body-mind':

4   *Performer Training for Actors and Athletes*

> Today I like to say "body-mind-world." You are not just body and mind, you are in the world, and I think it's important to acknowledge all the voices that come to us through the media, to interpret the information, to try to understand how the information is formed and how we can relate to what is happening, how we get our impressions. We bring our rational mind into play with our physical sense of response to all that information. I try to work with all that in a kind of stream of consciousness way because I don't want to be didactic or to pretend I have the answers but more to open a window on my questions [...].
>
> (quoted in Steffen 2012)

My conceptualization of bodyworld attempts a radical step further than Forti's 'body-mind-world' because the latter is still rooted in the human-centric outlook of an 'I' and its 'stream of consciousness way'. With bodyworld, the constitution and ontology of that 'I' is interrogated, revised, and expanded to include the involvement of the non-human, be that the natural world, other species, objects, clothing, equipment, or technology (Camilleri [2020] 2022: 157).

Understood in this way, therefore, 'bodyworld' indicates *a state of relational being with and in the world* while the plural 'bodyworlds' refers to *specific instances* of that state. The bodyworld writing these words (i.e. my relation with the world and the ensuing behaviour and experience) differs from my bodyworlds when I am in the theatre studio or when running a marathon. Although in principle this applies also to bodymind, the plural form ('bodyminds') is never deployed, precisely because the implication is that there is only one, singular, human-centred state or condition of bodymind. To speak of a 'performer's bodyminds' makes the shift from psychophysicality to post-psychophysicality, i.e. it acknowledges the diversity of relationalities with the non-human that impinges upon, conditions, and indeed constitutes the human. In this respect, then, the concept of bodyworld is more inclusive and explicit compared to bodymind (Camilleri 2020a: 26). It is important to emphasize that 'the post-psychophysical is not "anti-psychophysical" but "psychophysical+", i.e. a psychophysicality to a wider and deeper degree' (Camilleri 2019: xxii).

In an article about the kind of bodyworlds that characterize puppet and material performance (Camilleri [2020] 2022), the concept is further developed in terms of the so-called '3As', i.e. bodyworld as mind–body–world *assemblage*, whose constituent components offer a number of possibilities or *affordances*, some of which are transformed into performance material (ranging from body techniques to deployment of technologies to production logistics) and which come to function as *actants* (Latour 2005),

Introduction

that is, as *active elements* in the resultant multi-sourced output and that overlap with other socio-cultural networks. An example of the latter are the connections between the network–assemblages of theatres, public transport, and contracted cleaning services that enable practitioners to access and use a studio space for training and rehearsing (Camilleri 2019: 4–5).

The 3As are not discreet entities but formulations of the same phenomenon with affordances marking the *potential* and actants the *actualization* of the assemblage reality. The sequential relationship between the 3As is arbitrary. Affordances are dependent on the component elements in assemblages, and yet those same assemblages are possible only because the affordances of the constituent components enable them to come together. The same applies to the socio-cultural actants that are as *integral to* as they are *emergent from* the affordances of assemblages. The sequence adopted – assemblages, affordances, actants – is the consequence of patterns of thought in the West, which conceive of the visible-tangible body-assemblage as a *starting* point, i.e. an origin possessing capacities/affordances that are subsequently actualized, and which then act on the world around. An alternative sequence can conceive of the bodied assemblage as the *arrival* point that socio-cultural forces make possible through the coming together of properties/affordances.

The value of the 3As lies in their provision of an analytical base from which to approach elusive aspects of human embodiment such as cognition, affect, and agency. Although the 3As do not resolve such issues, they go some way in contextualizing them in three principal ways. First, the 3As serve to *situate* these phenomena theoretically. Second, this theoretical parsing facilitates the pragmatic *concretization* of these phenomena via exemplifications from practice, precisely in terms of constituent elements, their interactions and effects. Third, the practical specificities unearthed by the 3As suggest ways of intervening and *taking action*, i.e. how one approaches, prepares, and trains such aspects in practices like those that concern us here, namely sports as well as aesthetic performance like theatre and dance. Accordingly, the following section considers the fundamental but often overlooked example of *where* such practices take place, specifically by focusing on different implications of indoor and outdoor performances. For exemplification purposes, the emphasis is placed on the natural world even if, as noted earlier, bodyworld also includes the technological.

Bodies in the Open

The qualities of enacted presence, of *Umwelt* being, that the surrounding environment plays in sports brings out in sharper relief certain dimensions that are dormant, subdued, or otherwise concealed in many manifestations of aesthetic psychosomatic practice. I am referring to the dominant tendency to present theatre, dance, and other aesthetic performances indoors. *Performer Training Reconfigured* opens with a thought experiment that highlights the material features of a typical theatre or studio space in the twenty-first century (Camilleri 2019: 1–4). From the architectural features of the space, to the various technologies installed (including light, sound, ventilation, and other systems), to the equipment available (including training mats), all are part of the *assemblages that shape* (in constraining and facilitating) a practice.

The quantity and quality of the constitutive elements in such spaces varies according to the institutional, professional, or amateur status of the venue, which is accompanied by other assemblages that connect and feed into each other, such as the cleaning of the space and maintenance of equipment (e.g. with no working lights and access to sunlight no practice is sustainable). These socio-cultural actants, which mark components that play an active role in an assemblage (Bennett 2010: viii), impact the practice in a direct albeit at times invisible manner. For example, the responsibility in non-institutional contexts to clean and maintain one's own work space develops a different relation to the world, contributing an added dimension to the individual's work upon herself (Camilleri 2009: 30). However, irrespective of institutional or independent affiliation and save for exceptions that prove the rule, we are dealing with indoor spaces that are sheltered and have electricity as a bare minimum. As such, these are sealed spaces (some more hermetically than others) from the natural or urban environment that surrounds them and, therefore, from the world they seek to (re)present.

The overwhelming experience of aesthetic performance is framed and constricted by the ambient conditions of indoor spaces that, notwithstanding differences in design and features, are similar regardless of the productions on stage, especially if one frequents as spectator or operates as performer in the same venue. From the odours, colours, and textures of the place, to the quality of the air, sound, and lighting, to the feel of the chairs and of oneself in that environment, what drama occurs on stage takes place in the perception and imagination of the quasi-disembodied spectator via the abilities of the performers, technicians, and designers to transport the individual anywhere but the present space–time. This explains in part the appeal of immersive, site-specific, and even open-air performances that, at least in this regard, offer a richer *corporeality* (a *body-reality* as emergent from one's physicality and the surroundings' materiality) than merely sitting down in the semi-darkness of the same venue.

It is not a coincidence that a twentieth-century movement in theatre, aimed at investigating the actor's work and which has influenced more mainstream practices in the twenty-first century, is called a 'laboratory' (Brown 2019;

Introduction 7

Schino 2009). From Konstantin Stanislavski and Jacques Copeau to Jacques Lecoq and Eugenio Barba, from Ariane Mnouchkine to Anne Bogart and others, in seeking to limit variables and other distractions with the objective of facilitating and enhancing the practitioners' psychophysical focus and their 'inner life' (Richards 1995: 26), the bare studio laboratories of Peter Brook's 'empty space' and Jerzy Grotowski's 'poor theatre' also had the effect of neutralizing the presence of the environment. On the other hand, it is also true that the location of many of these spaces marked a retreat or a 'geographical displacement' from the dominant conditions of their theatre milieux (Camilleri 2009: 27).

In the case of sports, specifically those that are required to be held outdoors, both performers and spectators are exposed to the elements, foregrounding a bolder bodyworld dimension in the event experience: not only in terms of being affected by climate conditions (e.g. you get wet when it rains and sweat or burn in the sun) but more so with regard to the effectivity and accuracy of the athlete's performance who, unlike the indoors actor or dancer, needs to consider such things as rainfall, the direction and force of the wind, the varying textures and inclinations of the ground, the shifting positioning of the sun and its reflections on surfaces, high or low temperatures, as well as the vocal and visual reactions of the audience. It is a performance, therefore, that also happens to one's body as it reacts to and, at high levels of mastery, synchronizes and fuses with the elements of the world. Although no one performance, whether aesthetic, athletic, or in daily life, is exactly like another, this holds particularly true in scenarios where the natural environment plays its unscripted role. Conversely, with an indoors theatre, the 'environment' can be as scripted as the roles of actors in text-based drama – even more than that, it can be technologically *programmed* on cue.

Reference has already been made to instances of aesthetic practices that transcend conventional theatre-based spaces. These include ecosomatics that combine dance with ecological consciousness, like Helen Poyner's and Sandra Reeve's movement work in natural environments. Similarly, some currents in theatre history like Grotowski's paratheatre, Odin Teatret's 'barters' (Watson 2002: 94–6), and Gardzienice Theatre Association's 'expeditions and gatherings' (Allain 1997: 31–5; Hodge 2010b: 272), pushed the boundaries of 'theatre' in their practice of travelling, encountering people, and exchanging performances and experiences, usually in natural surroundings or non-theatre spaces. Moreover, contemporary genres like site-specific performance in urban settings also take place away from conventional theatre spaces that, in defamiliarizing one's expectations and experience of place, sensitize the participants to new bodyworld realities. Notwithstanding these performance externalizations of the practice, however, much of the actual training occurs primarily indoors, which is unlike a crucial characteristic in most sports that can only be practised outside.

An apposite example of outdoors aesthetic performance – perhaps even more than the Elizabethan open-air amphitheatres – is Ancient Greece, especially as woven within the fabric of other assemblages and socio-cultural actants. This includes the architectural and geographic features of the earlier theatres that were generally (but not exclusively) located away from the city, dug and carved out in the hills, open to the weather with natural light and acoustics, and, before the *skene* (or scenic space) started being constructed and elaborated, facing natural panoramas (Sokolicek et al. 2015; Bay et al. 2021). It is not a coincidence that, in the setting of the civic/religious rituals and ceremonies of the time, theatrical performances (which also included dance and music) were complemented by athletic competition. Writing about 'drama in dialogic Athens', Zarrilli notes that:

> religious rites often included competitions in honor of the gods, best exemplified in the well-known pan-Greek Olympic games (from 776 B.C.E.), held in honor of Zeus every four years following the summer solstice. Young male competitors trained for thirty days in foot and chariot racing, boxing, wrestling, *pankration* (martial arts), discus, and javelin – all of which contributed to military preparedness.
>
> (Zarrilli 2010: 60)

Other religious celebrations included the days-long Dionysian festivals, held annually in honour of the god of fertility and winemaking Dionysus, where the theatrical dramas were first performed:

> They were staged ultimately in a large outdoor amphitheatre, seating 10,000–15,000, located near the temple of Dionysus. The temple and the theatre were just below the Acropolis, the promontory at the center of Athens that served as both a stronghold and center of public life. […] the Great Dionysia began with a raucous procession […] followed by sacrificial rituals, civic ceremonies, and competitions in dithyrambs – choral songs and dances – and competitions of tragedies and comedies.
>
> (Zarrilli 2010: 61)

In such a context, aesthetic and athletic performance was 'ecological' not only in being closer to the natural environment but also in the sense that it was integrated within the broader community, encompassing social and cultural movements that were inseparable from religion and politics.

Introduction 9

Although there are various instances where sports are held indoors, and therefore the quality of bodyworld experience can be as framed or conditioned as in a theatre or dance studio, athletic practices like speed or endurance running and distance or height jumping also bring the physical environment to the fore by stretching the individual's psychosomatic capacities to the limits in terms of gravity, force (physical exertion), aerodynamics of movement and form, and similar aspects. The caveat bears reiterating that although indoor aesthetic and sport practices still relate to the 'world' of enclosed spaces and possess their specific bodyworlds, this section's focus on the ecological dimension of the outdoors highlights *important characteristics* of that experience. For example, the fact that humans can only partly mitigate but not fully control natural phenomena like the weather foregrounds bodyworld relationalities as well as the capacity and skill of the athlete/performer to manage the situation.

The broad brushstrokes of my argument in this section highlight the active role that the environment plays in open-air performance with the aim of exposing certain bodyworld relationalities that are obscured or overlooked in conventional understandings of aesthetic psychosomatic practice. The athlete's 'coupling with real-world scenarios' and her 'skillful engagement with the environment', which contribute to her sensorimotor know-how and 'adaptive intelligence' (Cappuccio 2019: xxvii, xix), can be something that theatre and dance learn more about from sports. To develop the picture with finer brushstrokes, the following section deals with affordances in sports from the perspective of embodied cognition.

ii. Bodyworld Affordances in Sports

Affordances in Action

An ecological approach to cognition conceives of *skilled behaviour* in terms of its *emergence* from the *constraints* of a combined *performer–environment* (P–E) system. This marks a more holistic perspective than a representational model based on an internal centralized controller that operates on the matching of mental patterns.

Constraints in an ecological P–E assemblage involve the physics (matter, energy, motion, and force) of the environment, the biomechanics of the body, the perceptual (and thus emotional) processing of body–environment interaction, as well as the specific demands of a task (Araújo et al. 2019: 537). Behaviour *emerges* from these constraints through processes of attunement and calibration, with the former signalling the *capacity* to perceive the state of play in an event, and the latter involving the actualization of possibilities in a given situation through the adaptation and scaling of *action*. As such, *capacity* and *action* constitute skill, which extends in range and faster reaction times with practice and experience. On such an ecological account, therefore, 'behaviour' is always already *constrained behaviour coupled with the environment*. A focus on affordances offers a fruitful approach to unpack some implications for skilled performance in psychosomatic processes like those of sports and aesthetic practices.

Referring to every 'separate decision' in sporting activities like sailing as functionally connected with all the other choices an individual makes (precisely because they emerge from dynamically evolving performance events like match-race regattas), sports psychologist Duarte Araújo, motor learning scientist Keith Davids, and philosopher of science and cognition Patrick McGivern argue that: 'This process of decision making ([e.g.] the selection of a path to the optimal starting point) clearly cannot be based on mental comparisons between optimal and actual states represented internally, because they emerge under the interaction of constraints such as an adversary's actions, wind changes, ocean currents, and personal preferences' (Araújo et al. 2019: 541). Araújo's research on expertise and decision making in sports led him and various colleagues to investigate what they term an event's 'landscape of attractors', i.e. stable variables in ongoing P–E interactions that frame behaviour and enable skilled solutions. As exemplified in the reference to sailing, which is typical of other sports (especially if held outdoors and involving simultaneous competitors), this landscape of opportunities presents evolving possibilities for action. It is with these *dynamic attractors*, which emphasize 'performer-environment reciprocity', that an understanding of affordances can be aligned (Araújo et al. 2019: 559–60).

Initially formulated by psychologist James J. Gibson (1904–1979), the theory of material affordances involves what the environment enables humans to do:

> The *affordances* of the environment are what it *offers* the animal, what it *provides* or *furnishes*, either for good or ill. [...] I mean by it something that refers to both the environment and the animal in a way that no existing term does. It implies the complementarity of the animal and the environment.
>
> (Gibson [1979] 2015: 119, emphasis in the original)

The theory states that the world is perceived not only in terms of shapes and spaces but also of object, terrain, and texture possibilities for action

Introduction

(Gibson [1979] 2015: 122–9). As such it is a theory of perception and action that signals a close connection between setting and organism, habitat and inhabitant, and, in our case, environment and performer.

In his introduction to the *Handbook of Embodied Cognition and Sport Psychology* (2019), cognitive philosopher and philosophical psychologist Massimiliano L. Cappuccio underlines the impact of Gibson's theory on sports and performance psychology. He argues that following Gibson, 'much of human performance—its physical and dynamic properties, with the possibilities, impossibilities, trajectories, and timing of limb movements—are determined primarily by the physics and biology of human anatomy [...], and only secondarily by the processes of perception, planning, and control' (Cappuccio 2019: xxii). Part VI in Cappuccio's edited volume, dedicated to 'Affordances and Action Selection', offers a comprehensive picture of the kind of theoretical and practical insights that an ecological focus on affordances provides, including with reference to assemblages/couplings and socio-cultural conditioning. The rest of this middle section of the Introduction weaves a literature review style of discussion that takes its cue from Cappuccio's Part VI to shed light on affordances in athletic and aesthetic performance.

Cognitive scientists and philosophers Wayne Christensen and Kath Bicknell identify three key claims in the Gibsonian account of affordances: '[1] *Affordances are action possibilities.* Thus, a cup affords grasping and a chair, sitting. [2] *Perception is primarily concerned with affordances.* Thus, Gibson says, "what we perceive when we look at objects are affordances, not their qualities. [...]" [3] *Affordances are perceived directly rather than represented*' (Christensen and Bicknell 2019: 602, emphasis in the original). Thus conceived, affordances are relational and action-relevant properties of the performer–environment assemblage, which includes not only the natural world but also tools, equipment, and technology. Regarding the last, Christensen and Bicknell highlight the role played by affordance perception in equipment design and its selection by individuals, referring to examples about how new bicycle technologies and rock climbers' shoes enable users to perceive and calibrate their decision making and behaviour (2019: 613).

In the light of this section's opening remarks about skilled behaviour, therefore, affordances can be viewed as emerging dynamically from the constraints of an evolving event. The dynamism of the situation also affects the stability and attraction of affordances, which fluctuate as new variables emerge (e.g. changes in weather) or are introduced (e.g. different equipment). The reciprocally (in)forming dynamic at play in affordances and their selection is evidenced by the fact that the quantity and quality of affordances are 'only accessible to individuals with the necessary skills to act on them':

12 *Performer Training for Actors and Athletes*

For example, where one soccer player with an excellent passing ability may perceive an opportunity to play a long pass to a teammate, another player who is highly skilled at running with the ball may perceive an opportunity to dribble past an opposing defender. Thus, sport people interact with a surrounding environment through skilled engagement with the concrete affordances that a specific environment offers them because of their unique skills.

(Araújo et al. 2019: 567–8)

This direct relation between perception processing and technical skill is at the root of the discussions developed in Parts I and II of this book, both as concerns the mental/physical capacities of athletic and aesthetic performers, as well as with regards to the role played by sensory and emotional feelings in these scenarios. In both instances, the mediating part played by the environment as foregrounded by affordances is of fundamental importance, hence my insistence on *bodyworld*.

Intentionality in Affordance

In their contribution to Cappuccio's volume, cognitive and sports scientists Andrew D. Wilson, Qin Zhu, and Geoffrey P. Bingham present a 'task-dynamical approach' to affordances that develops Gibson's theory by focusing on the kinetic and motor properties of athletes, specifically with reference to distance and accuracy throwing. The authors argue that, within a performer–environment task in sports, the 'language of dynamics provides all the elements required to describe the components, the organization of those components [...], the form of the change over time (the kinematics), and the forces that caused that particular motion (the kinetics)' (2019: 583). Wilson et al.'s approach to dynamics offers specific and additional insight into the nature of affordances. For example, their model brings to the fore a vital aspect of body–world interaction, i.e. the mediating energy media (such as the optic and acoustic arrays) that enable the perception of these otherwise inaccessible dynamics that are consequently offered as affordances. Since the energy media are exactly that, a *medium*, one important implication for behaviour concerns the scaling (or calibration) of action.

Consider, for instance, how calibration is conditioned by even the simplest of technology that, incidentally, also illustrates the prosthetic relationship with the world mentioned earlier: sunglasses enable the wearer to filter the 'blinding' information from the optic array in events like sailing and skiing that amplify the sunlight as it reflects off the sea and snow respectively. Such 'filtering' enables the individual to calibrate their resultant actions. Wilson

Introduction

et al.'s chapter, which deals with the affordances of throwing in sports, considers the processes of attunement and calibration in perception and action. Here, *attuning* involves visual and tactile information about the size–weight relation of the object being thrown, while *calibrating* requires which specific kinetic or effort variables to apply (2019: 588). Such mediation as provided by one or a combination of energy media constitutes one of the constraints that influences skilled behaviour and its intentionality.

Araújo, Dicks, and Davids view a skilled athlete's attunement to sources of information about oneself and the environment in terms of *decision making* that integrates 'intentions, actions, and perceptions' (2019: 559). They highlight an alternative conception of *intention* that accompanies a perspective of affordance. This is of direct relevance to the present book, concerned as Part I is with mental activity vis-à-vis bodyworld cognitions, attentional focus, and planning, and Part II with intentionality and affectivity. Their account of *intention as the selection of affordances* comes with a number of implications. Two such intention-as-selection cases identified by Araújo, Dicks, and Davids (2019) are worth outlining.

First, 'exploratory actions' (2019: 565), which are not performed with a specific intention in mind but with the purpose (or *intention*) of *finding an intention* in the emerging landscape of affordances during an evolving training or game situation. This kind of exploratory behaviour is connected to the richer information that movement makes available as opposed to a static perspective. While novices may engage in exploratory actions to search for existing options (i.e. configurations of play for which they have trained and can reproduce), more expert athletes tend to *create* them, for example, by forcing opponents to certain decisions, in which case the 'exploration' can overlap with feints intended to deceive the adversary. Another aspect of expert exploratory action concerns novel one-time solutions afforded by split-second reaction times. Creative improvisations of this kind in athletic and aesthetic performance are discussed in greater detail in Chapter 6.

Second, the 'nested dynamic state of organization' of a selected affordance refers to 'behavioral sequences' (Araújo et al. 2019: 566), i.e. the interconnection of actions – and therefore of intentions – in a task structure. By way of a concrete illustration, the 'nested dynamic' in a triple jump involves the three main actions of hopping, skipping, and jumping (which are in turn linked together within a running sequence), as well as the stances and movements that enable these individual actions, such as afforded by the traction of the ground, the athlete's footwear, and movement style. Nested affordances, therefore, do not necessarily require the activation of an internalized centralized controller that pre-determinedly 'intends' each action but often rely on expert automaticity as presented at various points in this book (see Chapters 1, 2, and 6).

The idea discussed in the previous section about the accessibility of affordances to individuals with the skills to actualize them can be extended to include skilled intentionality as part of the equation. In other words, and at the risk of labouring the point, skilled action emerges from the (skilled) intentionality of (skilled) perception in the (skilled) attunement of the P–E assemblage. This (skilled) behaviour is actualized through the calibration process of scaling. For example, it was found that:

> experienced goalkeepers scaled the timing of their actions relative to their agility when attempting to save penalty kicks. The more agile the goalkeeper, the later the diving action was likely to be initiated. [...] the slower goalkeepers who moved earlier exploited kinematic information from the penalty taker's action that led to a fewer number of saves and a greater likelihood of being deceived.
>
> (Araújo et al. 2019: 574)

This example illustrates a clear case of how perception attunement conditions calibration as a combination of spatial affordance-selection (where to jump) and temporal decision-taking (when to jump). The picture becomes more complex if the *penalty taker*'s calibration (of the intention to kick the ball) is considered in similar spatio-temporal terms, i.e. where, how, and when to kick the ball. The calibrated actions of both goalkeeper and penalty taker can be analysed from the lens of (1) 'exploratory actions', which are generally more evident in the goalkeeper's swaying movements aimed at distracting the penalty taker, but also present in the latter's lead-up to the kick, especially if involving unorthodox movements like a stuttering run up, and (2) 'nested dynamics', such as the quick reflex action when a goalkeeper changes direction in mid-leap or when she reaches out with an arm in the opposite direction of the leap.

iii. *Via Athletae* in Sports and Aesthetic Performance

The focus on *affordance in sports* as an aspect of a performer's *bodyworld* paves the way for this section's emphasis on *dimensions in aesthetic performance that can be aligned with skilled athletic behaviour*. The discussion, which adopts an expansive literature review style, is conducted mainly with reference to influential movements in twentieth-century theatre that have shaped or inspired body-based performance practices in the twenty-first century.

Introduction 15

The first name that probably comes to mind in a discussion about 'aesthetic athleticism' is that of French visionary, director, and actor Antonin Artaud (1896–1948). Although Artaud's story includes his search for the legendary long-distance Tarahumara runners in Mexico in 1936 (McDougall 2010: 19), as part of a quest for a more primeval relationship with nature and therefore with his own self (Krutak 2014: 29), my focus is his conceptualization of athleticism to mark a fundamental dimension in the actor's work. His notion of 'affective athleticism' refers to the actor who *feels* her movement in a broader and more holistic sense than the mainly biomechanical one discussed so far. The corporeality of Artaud's affective athleticism encompasses not only sensations and emotions but also a kind of all-consuming feeling and signification – *of being* – that transcends the theatre and that is potentially (and problematically, Jacques Derrida tells us) unmediated and unprocessed (Derrida [1967] 1978; Fortier 2016: 55–9).

Such a mode of perception and activity epitomizes a central maxim in twentieth-century theatre, i.e. a *training of the self* that does not only result in technical precision but informs an *ethical sensibility* within and beyond the theatre (Camilleri 2009; Camilleri 2015b). From Stanislavski, who explicitly used the phrase an 'actor's work on himself' for the title of his major book (Benedetti in Stanislavski 2008: xv), to others in his or from different lineages (like the French one delineated below), the narrative revolves around a re-working of the self. Accordingly, this third part of the Introduction puts forward the notion of *via athletae* (way of the athlete) to mark such a quality of being that is shared by aesthetic and athletic practices, irrespective of a body's form and abilities as long as there is consistency and depth of engagement.

A number of prominent theatre innovators and scholars in the twentieth century appear to have a predilection for boxing when writing about training and performance processes for actors (see also Evans 2012b). This may come as a surprise considering its combative nature because, despite being an Olympic sport with a long history dating back to Ancient Greece, it is 'for many too brutal and violent to be accepted as a sport' (Evans and Murray 2012: 141), let alone as aesthetic performance, regardless of its popular entertainment appeal. However, a recent article on aesthetic judgements in athletic performance sheds some light on the matter in distinguishing between two kinds of sports: '"aesthetic sports" (e.g., gymnastics, diving, figure skating; activities in which the aim cannot be specified in isolation from aesthetic concepts such as grace) and "purposive sports" (baseball, track and field; sports in which the aesthetic dimension is relatively unimportant as there are a huge variety of means by which one can achieve an end/one's goal)' (Toner and Montero 2020: 114). Boxing makes an intriguing case

16 *Performer Training for Actors and Athletes*

because, despite its antagonistic character, it combines the *purposive* with the *aesthetic*, i.e. when neither fighter achieves the 'purpose' of a knockout, the judges assess 'the quality of a boxer's performance; for example, cleaner punches, better defense' (2020: 114). From this angle, therefore, as a kind of liminal athletic/aesthetic practice, boxing and other combat sports like wrestling and martial arts have the potential of illuminating some aspects of *via athletae*.

Heart Athletes and Flying Acrobats

Artaud compared the actor with 'physical athletes' like boxers, wrestlers, runners, and high jumpers, specifically identifying the actor as 'a heart athlete' or an athlete of the heart ([1964] 2010: 93). Artaud's terminology highlights at once the similarities and the differences between actors and athletes. The similarities revolve around the 'anatomical bases' or the 'pressure points' in the body that enable the *movements* of boxers, sprinters, and other athletes *as much as* they facilitate the *emotional* sensibility of actors (93). Consequently, he speaks of the actor's 'affective musculature' that matches the 'bodily localization of feelings' (93).

The main differences between 'physical' and 'heart' athletes emerge in Artaud's focus on breathing as a crucial element in sports and theatre. He argues that 'an actor's body relies on breathing, while with a wrestler, a physical athlete, the breathing relies on his body' (Artaud [1964] 2010: 93). The emphasis on breathing allows Artaud to situate feeling in the patterns and dynamics of the body's movements, which in turn enables and constitutes a form of training 'in preparing [the actor] for his *craft*' (95, emphasis added).

Artaud's 'localization' – or training – of feeling also involves awareness, and thus the activation of a mental capacity: 'The main thing is to become *conscious* of these localizations of affective thought. […] The same pressure points which support *physical exertion* are also used in the emergence of *affective thought*' ([1964] 2010: 97, emphasis added). Artaud's actor, who 'thinks with his heart' (94), thus highlights the integration of physical, mental, and emotional dimensions as a pre-eminently human capacity that, on physiological and socio-cultural levels, has been lost or almost forgotten (99). However, this neglected quality of human embodiment can be reactivated, precisely through 'affective athleticism'.

Artaud's emphasis on training, therefore, is to teach the actor how to breathe, so that she knows how to feel (and thus also *what* to feel) and how to convey it. He hypothesizes a type of somatic/awareness training that focuses on the materiality and physicality – the *affordances* – of the human body

Introduction 17

as a way towards the im-material and the meta-physical: 'To know that an emotion is *substantial,* subject to the *plastic vicissitudes of matter,* gives him control over his passions' (Artaud [1964] 2010: 94, emphasis added). Artaud aligns such a formative practice for actors with athleticism, an athleticism that is not limited to muscular development but incorporates an emotional capacity that is assiduously cultivated through a practice of breathing, precisely an *affective athleticism* that renders it *aesthetic* for performers and audiences alike.

To refer to this kind or modality of athleticism, I take a leaf from Jerzy Grotowski's (1933–1999) 'poor theatre', specifically his principle of *via negativa* that marks an 'eradication of blocks' rather than 'a collection of skills' ([1968] 2002: 17), to propose a *via athletae,* a way of being athlete.

In an essay on Artaud entitled 'He Wasn't Entirely Himself', Grotowski admits that although Artaud left 'no concrete technique behind him' but visions and metaphors, he challenges theatre practitioners and students, especially with regard to the 'actor's art of extreme and ultimate action' ([1968] 2002: 118, 125). One dimension of this 'ultimate action' involves affective athleticism. Although still expressed in the language of metaphors, the emphasis on breath comes the closest to a practical approach when compared to other writings. Artaud's theoretical emphasis on affective athleticism can be grafted onto Grotowski's practical *via negativa* to yield a *via athletae* that underlines a material path towards an individual's optimal bodyworld performance. Such *individuality of optimization* in a training context is not predicated on a normative ideal body precisely because of the emphasis on the specificities of one's affordances.

Stephen Wangh's book *An Acrobat of the Heart: A Physical Approach to Acting Inspired by the Work of Jerzy Grotowski* (2000) captures one practical interpretation of the connection between Artaud and Grotowski. Wangh's metaphor of the actor as an 'acrobat of the heart' pays homage to Artaud's 'athlete of the heart', with the latter phrase featuring as an epigraph in the book along with two other quotations on acrobats and somersaults by Stanislavski and Grotowski respectively. The specific twist that Wangh gives to 'affective athleticism' concerns the 'moment of letting go' in performance:

> You can control each element of your preparation, you can concentrate on memories or images, you can tense or relax your body, and you can practice your gestures – but all this preparation is just that: preparation. […] Once the acrobat lets go of her trapeze, she again has choices to make. She cannot alter her momentum as she *flies,* but she can make use of it. She can choose to do a double flip, or she can choose to execute a

18   *Performer Training for Actors and Athletes*

twist. And the same is true for the actor. Once the emotion is *flowing* through you, you can choose to express it with a different tone of voice, or you can alter your timing, or your gesture pattern, or your blocking.

(Wangh 2000: 233, emphasis added)

The actor who 'flies' is not limited to technical perfection but involves a liberating Artaudian outlook that also 'flows' freely, unobstructed. Writing about Grotowski's corporeal exercises, which consist of a dynamic elaboration of static and introspective hatha yoga positions like headstands, shoulder stands, backbends, and rolls (Slowiak and Cuesta 2007: 139), Wangh warns about the dangers of the technical work becoming an end in itself, rather than a means to achieve one's acting goals. For him, the actor who flies is, first and foremost, an *actor* (rather than a technical acrobat), hence the necessity of concentrating on 'what the exercises do *for you as an actor*' (2000: 62, emphasis in the original).

The distinction between athleticism in sports and in aesthetic performance is fundamental to what ultimately separates the two disciplines, leading to different ontologies: whereas in the former, athleticism is an end in itself, with the individual striving to be(come) a better 'physical athlete', in the latter it is a means to an end, a *medium* of communication that relies on a credible 'heart athlete'. I return to this distinction towards the end of the book, in the context of aesthetic experience in athletic practice in Chapter 6, after surveying and investigating various aspects of the phenomenon in the intervening chapters. All this does not mean, however, that *via athletae* is available only to actors. As a 'way', it potentially applies to all spheres of life.

Action in Life

An instance of *via athletae*, one that overlaps with Artaud's milieu, can be found in Franco Ruffini's juxtaposition of boxing and acting processes in early twentieth-century France. Ruffini (1995) refers to 'the way of boxing' to shed light on the aspirations and methods of theatre innovator Jacques Copeau (1879–1949) and of his former student Étienne Decroux (1898–1991) who then went on to develop corporeal mime. Artaud operated in the same circles as Copeau and Decroux: he was influenced by the former via an apprenticeship with Charles Dullin (another student of Copeau), and he worked with Decroux on some projects, including directing him in at least one production (Leabhart and Chamberlain 2008: 11, 14).

The two other Frenchmen in Ruffini's account are Georges Hébert (1875–1957), a physical educator and trainer whose utilitarian 'natural method' in the military appealed to Copeau so much that he had it replace

Émile Jacques-Dalcroze's rhythmic approach in his school, and Georges Carpentier (1894–1975), the 'greatest of all "reformed" boxers' in the early twentieth century and whom Decroux identified as one of the 'driving images' of his mime (Ruffini 1995: 57, 61, 63).

According to Ruffini, the attraction of Copeau and Decroux to their sports counterparts revolved around the quality of behaviour they were seeking in their actors, that is, its *truth*: 'reality and not realism. In order for staged action to be true, i.e. fiction without lying, it must be *azione in vita* ["action in life"], i.e. real, and leaving aside any instance of realism' (1995: 54). In other words, Copeau and Decroux were fundamentally more interested in *function* than *style* in the generation of action: while *function* has an objective rooted in oneself-in-the-world and is commensurate with the affordances available, *style* shifts the emphasis onto display as an end justified only in itself, irrespective of the potential mismatch between an individual's ability and the exigencies of a task or situation. It is in this regard, therefore, and in its inherent biomechanical corporeality, that Decroux's mime prioritized function even as it developed a distinct style.

The fundamental principle that endeared Hébert's approach to Copeau involved his utilitarian method, which included the continuous training of eight exercises: 'walking, running, jumping, climbing, lifting, throwing, swimming and defending oneself' (Ruffini 1995: 60). These exercises were aimed at enhancing the student's psychophysical capacities in a holistic manner, as an integrated bodymind intent on fulfilling a purposeful task rather than targeting specific muscles, qualities, or dimensions for their own sake and at the expense of others.

Hébert's 'natural method' is often acknowledged as influencing the origins of parkour in France. This modern-day dynamic movement practice involves 'traversing obstacles in a man-made or natural environment through the use of running, vaulting, jumping, climbing, rolling, and other movements in order to travel from one point to another in the quickest and most efficient way possible without the use of equipment' (Bauer 2018). A crucial aspect of parkour, probably the dominant one in our twenty-first-century imaginary of the practice as relayed in photography and films, deals with the environment, i.e. the human body's flowing and adaptive movement in multi-levelled and multi-textured spaces.

The environmental setting was of central importance to Hébert, whose insistence on training outdoors recalls the earlier discussion about the specific bodyworld relationalities it generates: 'the utilitarian exercises help [the student] overcome obstacles that the environment itself places in his way. For example, he *jumps* over a fallen trunk that blocks the path of his walking; he *lifts* a rock that obstructs the course further on. He then proceeds

20   *Performer Training for Actors and Athletes*

to *throw* it into the thick vegetation, and so on' (Ruffini 1995: 61, emphasis in the original). Moreover, the level of difficulty, such as how far to run or how high/distant to jump, was determined by the student herself according to the principle of *auto-émulation* (or self-emulation), i.e. 'not against an abstract opponent or against absolute limits, but against [one]self' (Ruffini 2014: 81). In marking the desire and effort to improve oneself, *auto-émulation* emphasized not only a work on the self vis-à-vis the relation between objective, intention, and action, but also the *calibration* of perception–action that affordances require, as explained earlier.

Another early twentieth-century French connection between Hébert and theatre, also via Copeau and Artaud, concerns mime and movement pedagogue Jacques Lecoq (1921–1999), who began his professional life as a physical education instructor. Lecoq's knowledge of Hébert's 'natural method' increased after joining the theatre company of former Copeau student Jean Dasté (Evans 2016: 106). Mark Evans draws a compelling parallel between Hébert's 'natural gymnastics' and Lecoq's 'fundamental journey' exercise, which includes pulling, pushing, running, walking, lifting, and carrying:

> The engagement of the physical body of the student with the natural environment is a central part of the student's work with the [neutral] mask, and it is revisited repeatedly during that [first year] period of the training. This sense of a series of obstacles against which the students *test their creativity* is something that pervades the very ethos of [Lecoq's] school.
>
> (Evans 2016: 106, emphasis added)

Within Lecoq's pedagogical context, the 'test' marked by the tasks in the 'fundamental journey' functions in a manner that recalls Hébert's principle of *auto-émulation*. Even in Lecoq, therefore, the emphasis on performing concrete actions in a natural environment according to one's abilities resonates with Hébert's belief in an all-round formative process that encourages *azione in vita*. One aspect of this commensurability between capacity and affordances relates to the *effort* required to complete a task and thus to how it is manifested corporeally. Decroux offers a possible parallel to better understand this facet of *via athletae*.

The expressive embodied dimension of *via athletae* can be aligned with one of Decroux's primary 'styles or categories of acting': *l'Homme de Sport* or Man of Sport (Leabhart 1996, 2022: 124–69; Soum 1997: 17). Decroux's categories do not simply classify types and patterns of movement but involve a broader, even existential, stance or attitude that encapsulates an individual's state of being, and it is precisely this reflection that is incarnated by how

Introduction 21

one carries (i.e. *moves*) oneself. Corinne Soum (1997), one of Decroux's later students and assistants between 1978 and 1984, writes about the major categories of Man of Sport, Man in the Drawing Room, Mobile Statuary, and Man of Reverie. The distinguishing feature of Man of Sport concerns effort and its qualities. However, this category does not merely represent 'the sportive gesture, but of being inspired by it and of extracting a defined way of acting from this *condition of being*' (Soum 1997: 17, emphasis added).

Man of Sport as a category underlines Decroux's appreciation of sports as a quintessential human capacity. He admits that he 'always loved sports' because in it he saw the human struggle in a 'physical form' (in Leabhart and Chamberlain 2008: 63). Thomas Leabhart, another student and assistant of Decroux from 1968 to 1972, writes about the Man of Sport's 'C curve' configuration of the body or modality of movement. The 'C curve' is characteristic of 'sports activities (fencing, cycling, running, pitching a baseball, playing golf, basketball and ping-pong), as well as singing, floating in a bathtub, carrying packages, jumping rope, climbing stairs, squatting naturally as babies do, conducting an orchestra, yawning and pushing a refrigerator' (Leabhart 2022: 127–8). As a body position, the 'C curve' involves a 'low center of gravity and weighted movements' and can feature 'forward, backward, sideways and in rotation' (2022: 127, 136). The question of effort is of fundamental significance in corporeal mime because its interplays between weight and counterweight can have 'metaphysical' implications: 'A person wrestling with a burdensome idea or extreme emotion might resemble a person lifting a heavy weight' (2022: 135).

Decroux's categories of movement do not exist independently of each other in the sense that, as modalities of doing, they are subject to change and overlaps. Understood as such, Man of Sport marks an aspect of *via athletae* that is related to the manifested expression, and therefore also to its legibility by others. Decroux's admiration of Carpentier, who embodies the 'C curve' configuration of boxing, illuminates other – more immaterial – dimensions of *via athletae* that, while still rooted in 'physical form', put forward a being-in-the-*work* that reflects an ampler attitude of being-in-the-*world* that can be aligned with ethics.

Action in the Boxing Ring

The mid-nineteenth-century reform in boxing by the Marquess of Queensberry, which saw, amongst others, the use of padded gloves, timed rounds, ten instead of thirty seconds recovery when floored, plus the possibility of winning on points, changed the appearance and character of boxing from bare-knuckled bruisers to the leaner, agile, quicker, more

22   *Performer Training for Actors and Athletes*

precise, and psychologically intelligent athletes who aimed to deliver ten-second knockouts or win by points for more accurate punches (Ruffini 1995: 56–7).

Georges Carpentier epitomized the new breed of boxers (Decroux [1963] 1985: 14), particularly because he re-acted and adapted to the fighter in front of him: 'Carpentier boxed in a "natural" style, without unnecessary movements and sensational effects. [...] He would confine himself to doing the right thing at the right time, *nothing more and nothing less*. Though an entertainer, when he was in the ring, he made no concessions to theatrical displays' (Ruffini 1995: 58, emphasis added). Like Hébert's physical training, therefore, Carpentier's practice was guided by the exigencies of the situation, which, in the present account, can be re-read as the *affordances* that the athletes concretize according to their experience and skill.

Ruffini's analysis includes elements that were antagonistic to Hébert's and Carpentier's 'natural' methods, referring to *bodybuilding* and *hyper-competitiveness* as 'structural enemies' of their approaches (1995: 64; 2014: 82). From a utilitarian perspective, both *bodybuilding*, as the bulking of muscles for display, and *hyper-competitiveness*, as the taking on of unrealistic challenges doomed to failure, can be considered as ends in themselves: 'Neither one nor the other had its basis in conforming an action to an outcome that was simply objective and useful, as occurs in real life' (1995: 65). Both aspects were reflected in two major defeats that marked Carpentier's decline and eventual retirement in 1927. His loss against the heavier and younger Jack Dempsey in 1921 can be seen as a case of hyper-competitiveness, while the exhibition fight in 1922 that Carpentier was supposed to win against Battling Siki ended in defeat because he exaggerated the display of the punches rather than stuck to their 'utility' (66).

Although it marks a potential difference between sports and aesthetic performance, competitiveness per se is not the problem. While sports is inherently and explicitly *competitive*, the primary and final 'competitor' is the individual herself who is always striving to improve her performance. This fundamental premise in athletic activity parallels the actor's and dancer's work on oneself. Hébert's *auto-émulation* is, after all, a form of self-competition. Carpentier's 'doing the right thing at the right time', without any frills in the ring, is the result of his *preparatory* work on himself.

Conversely, aesthetic performance is inherently and explicitly *expressive* in the sense that, as a medium of communication and interaction, it essentially deals with the *organization of expression*, in training and public presentation. Although, as discussed in Chapters 1 and 6, an athlete's primary concern is with achieving a goal (winning a race, a 'personal best', etc.), the *organization* of one's optimal potential that *movement economy* entails inhabits a similar

Introduction   23

mechanism to aesthetics. For example, the calibration of perception and scaling of action that occurs in bodyworld relationalities during a sports activity marks one feature of this organization or 'aesthetic' in athletic behaviour.

The etymology of 'compete' from classical Latin (as distinct from the fourteenth-century French 'to be in rivalry with') is highly relevant to an appreciation of *via athletae*, for to capture the meaning of 'striving in common, together, or in company', it combines *com* 'with' and *petĕre* 'to strive' from the root *pet-* 'to rush, to fly' (Oxford English Dictionary; Online Etymology Dictionary). In other words, 'to compete' means *to fly with*, which is what the actor and athlete do in *via athletae* on various levels. Coupled with an ecological understanding of 'competition' as a struggle among organisms (Oxford English Dictionary), the concept typifies Decroux's Man of Sport, specifically as the effort of struggle and flight modulates between its sub-categories of the Man of Affliction's load-bearing and The Artisan's craft and ingenuity (Soum 1997: 18).

Ruffini's problem with excessive or hyper-competitiveness involves the unrealistic objectives situated beyond one's bodyworld, i.e. 'physical exercise to obtain exceptional performances and victory over one's opponents at all costs, and *not to improve oneself and raise one's limit*' (2014: 82, emphasis added). In other words, the placement of an individual *beyond* herself as signalled by the discrepancy between capacity and task requirements, thus defying reality in the inflation of bodyworld affordances. In Ruffini's reading, Carpentier's fights with Dempsey and Battling Siki exemplified two such instances of the separation between 'real' and 'fake' boxing.

And yet, as performance ethnographer Solomon P. Lennox observes in his work with amateur and professional boxers, it is difficult and problematic to 'differentiate between those elements which can be understood as the "real" sporting activity, and those which are "feigned" and theatrical' (Lennox 2012: 210). The relationship between boxing and entertainment that Lennox explores in current fighters is echoed in Carpentier, who performed as a film actor and a music hall entertainer, mainly to display his boxing skills (Ruffini 1995: 58). In these exhibition cases, Carpentier's 'functional' and 'real' boxing became, literally, a 'style' of acting.

To investigate the relationship between 'real' and 'theatrical' boxing, Lennox focuses on the kind of 'boxer-entertainers' trained in Brendan Ingle's (1940–2018) Wincobank gym (Sheffield, UK), which produced four world champions and other successful fighters. Ingle-trained boxers are often criticized for their 'theatrical' excesses, such as the unconventional antics of 1995–2000 featherweight world champion 'Prince' Naseem Hamed, which included 'spectacular ring entrances, his somersaults over the ropes at the start

24   *Performer Training for Actors and Athletes*

of each bout, and the amount of acrobatic flips and showboating he engaged with during each fight. Thus, he seemingly blurred the boundaries of what is "real" and "legitimate" sport, and that which is "feigned", performed, and theatrical' (Lennox 2012: 212). In his extravagant style, Hamed represented the flip version of Carpentier's 'nothing more and nothing less' approach to boxing. And yet, both were highly effective in their different ways as reflected in their successes in the ring.

Despite the different styles of Carpentier and Hamed, a subterranean connection can possibly be located in their preparation. Lennox reports that, apart from conventional boxing exercises such as mitt work and sparring, Ingle included dance-like movement patterns, acrobatic drills, and even singing in his training and punching routines. These 'idiosyncratic performance practices' were not so much added as incorporated into the daily training (Lennox 2012: 211). In other words, these supposedly extraneous exercises to boxing were 'holistically integrated', in the process also *combining in embodiment* the roles of athlete and entertainer in Ingle's vision (209). Considered as part of a daily practice, these 'theatrical' elements were not optional extras but key aspects that complemented, fulfilled, and enhanced the boxing formation of individuals.

According to Lennox's research, Ingle was interested in a rounder and fuller individual than a boxer as narrowly defined by the conventions of the sport. For him, the kind of 'performance' training that Lennox describes is not only 'central to the development of athletic ability' but also to life after boxing (2012: 211). As amateur boxer Matt Hunter acknowledges: 'Ingle's training practices enabled him to develop key social skills which he did not acquire through primary or secondary education. These skills *afford* the boxer with greater levels of independence outside of the confines of the boxing culture' (Lennox and Rodosthenous 2016: 153, emphasis added). In the current context, the choice of the word 'affords' takes on added significance that sheds light on the *immaterial dimension of affordances* that psychosomatic practices like boxing and theatre make available for their respective bodyworlds. That is, in *affording* a different form of perception, this kind of training enables decision making and action taking *also* in the (socio-cultural) world-out-there beyond the boxing ring.

Punches in the Face of Ethics and Reality

The immaterial dimension of skilled behaviour that accompanies certain instances of athletic and aesthetic performance can be aligned with a conception of ethics that Ruffini associates with the 'truth' of an action. In such instances, 'truth' conforms to 'reality' in life, i.e. not to the *stylistic manner* of an action but its *psychophysical matter* of execution. One possible bridge between this intersection of movement and ethics can be found in the concept and dynamic of *play*.

From this perspective, Ingle's fusion of athletic and aesthetic modes in his boxing approach was effective (on and off the ring) because the 'extraneous' and 'excessive' dancing, acrobatics, and singing foreground an attitude of *play* (sometimes even of *role-play* in the case of Hamed) that, as already discussed, *afforded* new solutions that could otherwise be missing in more discipline-specific training. Copeau wrote about 'specialist athletes' who, like other virtuosos (even in the theatre), 'overdevelop' certain aspects at the expense of others. This excess (or *'cabotinage'* as Copeau called it) hampers an individual's *'equilibrium of the heart* [....] in other words, their *character'*, once again connecting the 'muscular' with an ethical 'spirit' (Ruffini 2014: 83, original emphasis).

Conversely, a performer who 'flies' implies soaring above the constrictions of specialized and overdeveloped technique that, however effective, can become habitual and predictable and therefore lacking in *vita* (life/vitality). As a consequence, the richer and more open range that the mechanisms and dynamics of *play* afford is of crucial importance to theatre-makers, including for Copeau but in particular Lecoq who built his pedagogical improvisatory practice around it. Lecoq's *le jeu* (play) is discussed as a fundamental priming capacity for movement in Chapter 4, but here it suffices to outline a connection between sports and a mode of performing.

Lecoq's interest in sports is reflected in his school's first year Movement Analysis sessions (Evans 2016: 107; Lecoq [1997] 2002: 69, 94; Murphy 2019a: 6). These classes involve performing a sequence of twenty of the movements transmitted to them (Lecoq [1997] 2002: 15). As Evans observes, although many of these actions 'refer to or are representations of sporting activities' (like skating, rowing, punting, and discus-throwing), athletic precision per se is not the principal objective. The emphasis, rather, recalls the essence of sports as a *play* activity – a notion that is central to Lecoq pedagogy, not only in reflecting an individual's freedom and therefore her expressive capacity, but also, like Decroux's movement categories, as a metaphor for life. In this regard, Lecoq distinguishes 'movement' as physical motion from 'Movement with a capital "M"' as life more generally (Lecoq [1987] 2006: 81).

Referring to the presentations of the Twenty Movements, Evans argues that:

> it is through the *play of technique and sequencing* [of the selected movements] that the *student reveals him/herself*, demonstrating an ability to create through movement a sense of rhythm, space, weight and

26 *Performer Training for Actors and Athletes*

ultimately *emotion and meaning*. The student is encouraged to perform the movements *economically*, avoiding psychological explanations ([...]), so that the movements can serve as a form of reference point around which the student can *play imaginatively*.

(Evans 2016: 107, emphasis added)

This passage highlights a number of key elements in Lecoq's work, connecting technique, imagination, meaning, and identity/individuality with expressivity through play and efficient/effective behaviour. While the emergence ('revelation') of oneself through movement resonates with a broader ethical dimension, the accent on 'economical' performance parallels the preference of an action's function over its style that Ruffini identifies in Copeau and Decroux. A movement is 'economical' precisely when it achieves its objective efficiently, that is, without the inclusion of elements deemed extraneous to the task. And yet, in Ingle's gym, the play dynamics afforded by the non-boxing exercises appear to have been instrumental in accomplishing boxing purposes.

Ruffini associates work 'as occurs in real life' with 'an ethical profile' of actors who are 'open to what surrounds them and ready to respond. In a word, they are *in vita,* if to be *in vita* means precisely to understand, to capture external reality and to be able to react to it' (Ruffini 1995: 65, 68). Insofar as the individual engages with a deep practice of awareness and commitment that is not only formational (within training) but also transformational (beyond training), the 'ethical profile' of performers can manifest itself in different ways, from Lecoq's 'economical movement' to Ingle's 'theatricality' in boxing.

In a fuller account of the subject, Ruffini foregrounds the centrality of an ethical profile by means of the metaphor in the title of *Theatre and Boxing: The Actor Who Flies* (2014):

In order to fly, a human being must re-build his body. [...] Re-building the body means re-building the body's consciousness [...] achieving a perception other than the one imposed on us by society of a body chained to the ground. [...] The theatre is the place where bodies are re-built: and so the actor can fly.

(Ruffini 2014: 145)

In the final analysis, it is always a question of perception – of ethical insight as much as sensorial sight – that trained (re-built and re-*assembled*) bodies *afford*. When actualized, these *assembled* biomechanical and physiochemical

Introduction 27

affordances become socio-cultural *actants* that play a role in any given narrative, be it aesthetic, athletic, or in daily life, including the life-after-boxing qualities of Ingle's fighters. It is in this way that the immaterial dimensions of a material practice determine an ethical sensibility, thus revealing (or 'un-concealing' in the etymological sense of *alētheia*/truth) what can be viewed as 'ethical affordance'.

If actors have the capacity to be true and real in the theatre fiction they embody on stage, Ingle's boxers have the potential to be as true and real in their theatricality in the ring. However economical or functional its movement might be, the reality of a punch in the face in daily life is always already 'theatrical', larger than life, within the socio-cultural and *communitas* boundaries of human interaction. Conversely, the reality of a punch in the face *in a boxing ring* is not rendered less truthful because of any additional 'theatricality' it assumes in a dance routine or within a spectacularized context. Such a *mode* of 'theatricality' functions in a similar way to what in Chapter 2 is denoted by 'epistemic action', i.e. an indirect, scaffolded way of achieving an objective. According to the insider testimony of many of Ingle's boxers (Lennox 2012; Lennox and Rodosthenous 2016), what for outsiders passes as 'feigned' behaviour becomes a role comparable to the actor who flies.

Enduring Humanity

Among the drawings by Keigo that are evoked in the opening section of this Introduction, there are two that offer a solution for the embattled alligator who keeps falling short as he engages in various human activities, whether in sports, the performing arts, or daily life. One of these successful outcomes deals with a yoga-like stretch position of touching the floor in front of his toes with the legs held straight. The other instance portrays a balancing act on one leg on a balloon ball. In both cases, the alligator accomplishes the task in an alternative way to the typical human approach. Instead of touching the floor with the fingertips, the alligator does so with the end of his snout while keeping the recommended form for the legs and back, thus achieving the stretch objective of the exercise. And instead of balancing on one leg with arms spread sideways, he extends them backwards to counterweight his forward projecting snout. Very tellingly, the balancing act in Keigo's cartoon recalls Decroux's 'C curve' body configuration of the Man of Sport, which, in expressing effort and struggle, provides an apt metaphor for the alligator's lot in the Anthropocene.

28 *Performer Training for Actors and Athletes*

The alligator's effective solutions mark *ways of doing* that are appropriate to the affordances of his particular body. Like Hébert and Carpentier, the alligator's objective is commensurate with the capacities and abilities of *his* – not someone else's – body. Consequently, in *being true* to his body-in-the-world, the alligator marks, first, a *way of being* and, second, a fundamentally *ethical stance* – a 'truth' – towards oneself and/in the world. Both way of being and ethical sensibility, which converge in and emerge from the alligator's skilled behaviour, reinforce the suggestion of an immaterial dimension in the work. In this Introduction, an individual's *corporeal truth* to the *material reality* she inhabits has been aligned with a modality I have called *via athletae*. As presented here, this embodied 'truth' and environmental 'reality' are not idealized or rhetorical constructions but directly linked to an understanding of bodyworld affordances.

Via athletae is not a method or route. In serving as a quest of the self that, through training, is also a re-making of the self, *via athletae* marks a *journey* that is specific to the individual, irrespective of one's body shape or condition and of the discipline in which one operates. Writing from experience as an athlete and sports coach, Matt Fitzgerald speaks about a 'journey of self-becoming' that is available to those 'who accept the challenge […] that leads toward full realization of inner potential' (Fitzgerald 2016: 265). A similar journey can be located in aesthetic performance. Writing about Artaud but also illuminating his own position, Grotowski observes that: 'an actor reaches the essence of his vocation whenever he commits an act of sincerity, when he unveils himself, opens and gives himself in an extreme, solemn gesture' ([1968] 2002: 124). The 'act of sincerity' in the 'essence' of an actor's work again underlines a *way of being* oneself.

The nature of such a self-consuming and self-transformational journey is reflected in the more measured words of practitioner-scholars Mark Evans and Simon Murray, who round up their editorial for a special issue of *Theatre, Dance and Performance Training* dedicated to 'Sport' with reference to 'the extent to which both athletes and performers commit fully, both physically and emotionally, to training processes that ultimately challenge and change them in significant ways'. It is precisely this re-working and transformational potential of the trained self that takes 'us outside of ourselves and at the same time deeper into what it means to be ourselves' (Evans and Murray 2012: 144).

One manifestation of the transformational effect of this journey is a trained body, but that is only a part of the story, for *via athletae* does not privilege a specific body type. In fact, what in the socio-cultural imaginary constitutes a normative 'athletic body' does not exist per se when considering the different bodies of Kenyan marathoners, heavyweight boxers, Paralympians, netball

Introduction 29

players, ageing golf professionals, and other athletes to name but a few. Indeed, one consequence of a way of doing/being that focuses on somatic dimension *is* a trained body. Equally undeniable, however, is that various sports require or generate typical bodies for that activity, which applies to varying degrees in dance as well as in many spheres in life, with certain skills and trades affecting bodies, from manual to factory workers to sedentary office jobs.

The case of actors may well be an exception that proves the rule: individuals with differently shaped bodies in traditional theatre or film can embark on or traverse their own *via athletae* as much as those with more 'athletic' bodies in physical theatre. (As for the predilection that exists for certain body types on stage and screen in terms of race, size, age, and gender, this is something that reflects socio-cultural biases rather than a physiological requirement for or consequence of acting, which is the point here.) In this context, then, a body in *via athletae* may be 're-built' – even 're-sculpted' – in various ways. To denote the athletic/aesthetic spectrum of trained bodies I propose the neologism 'aesthletic' to capture the particular and sometimes also peculiar qualities generally associated with notions of 'grace', 'beauty', or simply 'form' that worked-upon bodies possess or acquire in a *via athletae*.

What distinguishes *via athletae* from other ways of being is a modal emphasis on physical engagement, which also marks an intensified engagement with the world's materiality. Pushing something to its limit, conceptually and physically, is not exclusive to endurance athletes. Grotowski writes about Artaud's requirement of the actor's 'extreme, solemn gesture' ([1968] 2002: 124). According to Ingemar Lindh (1945–1997), another former student and assistant of Decroux, pushing an exercise or a concept to an extreme enables the examination of *what it really is* (Lindh 2010: 76; Camilleri 2008c). Decroux's development of corporeal mime as an independent artform came as a result of pushing to an extreme one of his teacher's (Copeau's) training exercises, i.e. silent improvisation aimed at making the actor's body more expressive (Barba [1993] 1995: 109–10).

In this section, Ruffini's reference to the 'truth' and 'reality' of an *azione in vita* has been contemplated in the context of a *way of being* associated with athleticism. Endurance sports go one step forward, presenting us with what six-time Ironman winner Mark Allen calls 'raw reality'. This is when, in the words of Fitzgerald, 'an inner curtain is drawn open, *revealing a part of you* that is not seen except in moments of crisis. And when your answer is to keep pushing, you come away from the trial with the kind of *self-knowledge* and self-respect that can't be bought' (Fitzgerald 2016: 261, emphasis added). Like Artaud's impossible vision of an unmediated experience for an actor and her spectators, such 'raw reality' makes manifest a 'raw truth' that is as divested of form as is humanly possible in its immediacy. As such, determination, persistence, and stamina – even when they feature in non-athletic (and more cerebral) activities – suggest other dimensions of *via athletae*.

Endurance sports is not a version of hyper-competitiveness. On the contrary, it can be viewed as pushing Hébert's 'natural approach' to the extreme of one's bodyworld affordances. Accordingly, it shines a light on aspects that may be obscured in other athletic and aesthetic practices, hence the inclination in the following chapters to reference it, especially in the context of long-distance running. As Vybarr Cregan-Reid, professor of English and environmental humanities with specialized interests in biomechanics and sports science, points out in the title and text of his book on running, it is what 'makes us human' (2016). In quasi-Artaudian words that resonate with 'affective athleticism', he tells us that:

> Navigating our way through a landscape changes the means by which we may experience it. If our heart-rate is raised, if endorphins are flooding our system, if our veins and capillaries have dilated to increase the flow of oxygen to the muscles and the brain, if we can feel the microtexture of the earth changing beneath our feet, the world becomes a different place. The world stops being a picture for us to gawp and yawn at, and *the relationship between our insides and its outsides becomes a dynamic one* [...]. *Running reminds us that our bodies and the world are made of the same stuff.*
>
> (Cregan-Reid 2016: 62, emphasis added)

Performer Training for Actors and Athletes tackles such phenomenological and physiological dimensions of bodyworld with the aim of telling us something about ourselves, not only as aesthetic and athletic performers but, like Keigo's alligator, the extent to which 'my presence', 'my intention', 'my imagination', and 'my agency' are indeed *mine* in the world.

Part I

Mind Games

1

I Perform, I Think: Bodyworld Cognitions

Haruki Murakami (b. 1949), the international bestselling and award-winning novelist, is also an experienced marathon runner. He writes about his relationship with long-distance running in *What I Talk About When I Talk About Running* (2008). A memorable section in this memoir concerns the ultramarathon he ran in 1996 at the age of 47. An ultramarathon is any race longer than the 42.2-km (26-mile) distance of a marathon. Murakami managed to run the 100 km (62 miles) of the Lake Saroma Ultramarathon (Hokkaido, Japan) in eleven hours and forty-two minutes. His account of the event reads like a lifetime of sensations and emotions: from the pedestrian normality of the first 55 km (34 miles), to the gruelling middle section where his legs, in turmoil, 'had a mind of their own', to the rarefied existence beyond the 75-km (47-mile) mark, when he felt like his body had 'passed clean through a stone wall' and that he was on 'autopilot', detached from a sense of self (2008: 106–15). That's a lot of feeling for a day, including when he 'didn't think about anything [and] didn't feel anything'; all that mattered was the act of running: 'I run; therefore I am' (113).

Murakami's ultramarathon experience evokes the state of the performing body pushed to an extreme: movement, feeling, emotion, thinking, being, and the connections in between. This chapter focuses on the bodyworld of actors and athletes from the perspective of cognition, specifically as prompted and essentialized by thought processes during running. To this end, the chapter examines the 'mind' aspect of the body–world assemblage because, in the endeavour to shift the focus on to the somatic, the mental dimension is often overlooked, no doubt to compensate for the privileged position it has occupied in the West and that still conditions conceptions of the integrated body. This re-evaluation of the mind in somatic practice draws on insights from sports science and aesthetic performance.

Thinking About It

Murakami recounts that he is often asked what he thinks about as he runs. Although he claims that he does not 'think much', his list of random thoughts tells us that, paradoxically, he 'thinks' quite frequently when running, mainly

34   *Performer Training for Actors and Athletes*

about (1) the world and its impact on him (how cold/hot it is), (2) his own emotional state (how sad/happy he is), (3) past events and experiences (memories), and (4) very occasionally, 'ideas' for his writing (2008: 16–17). In addition to *a lot of feeling*, therefore, there also seems to be *a lot of thinking* going on when running. He elaborates: 'I run in a void. Or maybe [...] I run in order to *acquire* a void. [...] What I mean is, the kinds of thoughts and ideas that invade my emotions as I run remain subordinate to that void' (2008: 17, emphasis in the original).

To Murakami, a mental void implies lacking an organizing structure that gives meaning ('content') to what otherwise are 'random thoughts' and 'random memories'. However, running to 'acquire a void' in itself marks an objective, and as such is implicated in psychologies of motivation, aspiration, or even therapy, that in turn involve a cognitive process. While elite athletes and competitive amateurs endeavour to finish as high up in a race as possible, Murakami's interest 'to beat [...] the way you used to be' (2008: 10) also entails adjusting one's frame of mind (one's *thoughts*) in specific ways. Additionally, the quest for a void overlaps with another form of 'thinking', especially in the context of his primary occupation as a novelist. Although Murakami may 'hardly ever get an idea to use in a novel' when running, his decades-long running practice informs his writing at a subterranean level as evoked implicitly in (and explicitly by) his memoir.

The early sports training of physical theatre and mime teacher Jacques Lecoq provides a clue about the connection between physical and mental movement:

> My first introduction to [movement] was in stadiums and swimming pools, where I could enjoy the simple act of moving: the *body's extension* in throwing the discus, pacing my breath and stride in running races, that moment of suspension just above the bar in the high jump. These actions *expanded my mind* [...]. *My body remembers* all of this. I can recall doing a 1,500-metre swim where time gradually seemed to slip away and the steady rhythm of my front crawl helped me *solve a maths problem* that I had been set for homework.
>
> (Lecoq [1987] 2006: 96, emphasis added)

Murakami's thought-void can be juxtaposed with the sensations foregrounded in Lecoq's experience of physical activity: the young Lecoq did not think about anything except living the mo(ve)ment. The immersion in movement 'extended the body' and 'expanded the mind', leading to a kind of *corporeal thinking* marked by the 'body that remembers'. Even more illuminating, Lecoq connects this expansive corporeal thinking with the abstract and

Bodyworld Cognitions 35

sophisticated computation of a mathematical challenge. Something must have moved him at a deeper level: something related to perception (of one's body and/in the world) and its cognitive processing. Murakami's thought-void of 'I run; therefore I am' possibly impacts his novel-writing in subtle and complex ways that weave body–mind–world together, including thinking/writing *after* the act of running.

When Murakami went past the 75 km mark, he stopped trying to think: 'more precisely, there wasn't the need to try to consciously think about not thinking. All I had to do was go with the flow and I'd get there automatically. If I gave myself up to it, some sort of power would naturally push me forward' (2008: 112). This is reminiscent of theatre-makers like Jerzy Grotowski and Ingemar Lindh, whose '*via negativa*' and 'disinterested act' respectively marked a specific mental state that resulted in action almost in spite of oneself (Camilleri 2011: 306). For example: 'The requisite state of mind [in *via negativa*] is a passive readiness to realize an active role, a state in which one does not *want to do that* but rather *resigns from not doing it*' (Grotowski [1968] 2002: 17, emphasis in the original). The crucial difference may be that Murakami's void was induced by exhaustion, whereas in Grotowski, Lindh, and similar aesthetic performance practices the 'letting go' is prompted by choice. However, a closer inspection reveals substantial overlaps as illustrated by Thomas Richards during a 1984 intensive workshop with Grotowski:

> At first [...] I was mentally interpreting the songs. [...] Well, we danced for a long time, it seemed we must have been going for some hours, nonstop. After a certain point, as my physical exhaustion grew, my mind became tired and quiet: it was less able to tell my body how to interpret the song. Then for some short moments I felt as if my body started to dance by itself. The *body* led the way to move, the mind became passive.
> (Richards 1995: 22–3, emphasis in the original)

If anything, this tells us that the 'choice' aesthetic performers make to let go of their mental controller during performance is trainable and one way to do so is, precisely, through pushing oneself to the limits of physical endurance. It must be highlighted, however preliminarily at this point, that endurance is connected to repeatable actions, whether it is running, dancing, singing, or other forms of movement.

Of course, we are always 'thinking', even when, like Murakami and Richards, we do not 'consciously think' about it, which suggests that there are different forms of 'thinking'. When running, you think *about* running – including past the threshold that Murakami speaks about – it is part of the 'flow' and 'automaticity', the 'power' and 'nature' he mentions that

36   *Performer Training for Actors and Athletes*

pushes him forward in spite of himself because of his *readiness* to complete the task. The same applies to other performers, whether aesthetic or in daily life: at a fundamental but conscious level, every actor *knows* that she is acting a role or playing a score of actions. As such, because of this *knowing*, every actor is 'thinking about' acting when acting. The question, therefore, is not an existential *if* but a modal *how*. In Grotowski's case it involves an interplay between active and passive engagement, but an *engagement* (a 'readiness') nonetheless. Likewise, Murakami is never 'not knowing' that he is running. The current chapter is concerned with the nature of this 'knowing' and 'thinking'. As should be clear by now, 'thinking' is too broad a term to capture the specificities of the various types of cognitive processes and consequences evoked thus far. A primary aim of this chapter is precisely to identify more specific terminology to distinguish between the various cognitions that characterize the performing body.

Mind Mapping

A 2012 study by a group of sports psychologists sought to 'map the runner's mind' via real-time tracking technology (Quintana et al. 2012). A major objective of the experiment aimed to rectify the often-cited methodological limitations of retrospective recall and intermittent processes that are usually used to gather data about an athlete's cognitions *after* the event. For the purposes of the current chapter, however, rather than the technology itself (the software and ergonomic joystick that the participants interacted with while running), I am more interested in what it was deployed to identify, i.e. the researchers' classification and definition of 'cognitions':

> Cognitions were defined as the mental activities involved in acquiring and processing information [...] and consisted of four specific directions: *Images*: cognitions related to the mental representation in which the runner observes himself doing something. *Emotions*: content related to an affective state during the running session. *Sensations*: cognitions related to the subjective experience of feeling that resulted from stimulations derived from the physical effort of running. *Thoughts*: those that appeared during the running session but do not have to do with images, emotions or sensations.
>
> (Quintana et al. 2012: 591)

The overlapping qualities of these four categories, especially concerning sensorial and emotional feelings and their processing, does not make this

Bodyworld Cognitions 37

the sharpest of conceptualizations, but it is an instrument nonetheless that enables analysis. For all intents and purposes, cognitions are forms or qualities of 'thoughts' that are inflected differently according to their stage and location of development in the same bodyworld process. As discussed in more detail in Chapter 4 (see also Camilleri 2019: 147–53; Camilleri 2020a: 27–9), sensations, emotions, and their cognitive processing (such as visualizations and memories) can be situated on an experiential continuum that emerges from a body's interaction with the world. This chapter concentrates on cognition as an overall category for mental activity as 'thought' that occurs during athletic and aesthetic performance, i.e. as an illustration of body/mind/world.

Sports and exercise psychologists Noel Brick, Tadhg MacIntyre, and Mark Campbell present an updated model of attentional focus to better categorize cognitive processes and 'conceptualise all thoughts' by athletes during endurance events (2014: 107). They build on research stretching back to the late 1970s and 1980s that classified the cognition of marathon runners into *associative*, or the monitoring of sensory information typically linked with elite athletes, and *dissociative*, or the alienating of 'painful sensory input' connected with non-elite participants (Morgan and Pollock 1977: 390, 391, 399). More specifically, they develop Clare D. Stevinson and Stuart J. H. Biddle's classification of 'cognitive orientations in marathon running' (1998) that incorporated *internal* and *external* directions in *both* associative and dissociative categories. Previously, internal and external focus were often considered exclusively from each other (Brick et al. 2014: 109).

Brick et al.'s model is informed by a review of 112 studies that involve attentional focus variables in endurance exercise and performance. Their analysis deploys terms like *attentional focus* or *cognitive orientations* for cognitions that are 'not necessarily planned or deliberate', but reserves *strategy* for 'thoughts [that] are intentionally utilised to modify aspects of exercise performance' (2014: 108). With regard to associative aspects, Brick et al. extend Stevinson and Biddle's *internal association* category in two directions, distinguishing between *internal sensory monitoring* and *active self-regulation* to differentiate bodily sensations from thoughts related to technique. Concerning dissociation, they adopt Stevinson and Biddle's term *distraction* but fine-tune the inward/outward distinction by distinguishing between the *active distraction* of 'settings that demand active or directed attention (e.g. a busy urban street)' and the *involuntary distraction* of 'attractive stimuli (e.g. picturesque scenery)' (2014: 112; cf. Cregan-Reid 2016: 105–6, 109). A key development on Stevinson and Biddle is the placement of strategy thoughts. Traditionally considered as external association/monitoring, Brick et al. view it as an internal phenomenon, specifically as *active self-regulation*, arguing that: 'Although athletes may *outwardly monitor* environmental conditions or competitors, effective strategic decisions are ultimately based on one's own capabilities' that are actualized in terms of pacing and effort (2014: 112).

Brick et al.'s updated model of 'attentional focus dimensions during endurance activity' thus consists of the following categories, including some 'thought examples' as extracted from their article:

(1) *internal sensory monitoring*, e.g. effort sensations, breathing, muscle soreness, fatigue, perspiration, thirst, blisters;
(2) *active self-regulation*, e.g. running technique, cadence (i.e. steps per minute), relaxing (i.e. maintaining a relaxed state), pacing, strategy;
(3) *outward monitoring*, e.g. route, conditions (climate, environment, etc.), split times (i.e. time taken to complete a specific distance), distance information/mile markers, other competitors, water stations;
(4) *distraction*:
   a. *active distraction*, e.g. attention-demanding tasks like puzzles, attention-demanding environments like urban streets, intentional distraction, conversing, watching videos (when using a treadmill);
   b. *involuntary distraction*, e.g. unimportant scenery, attractive environment, spectators, other non-competitive runners, reflective thoughts (like philosophy, politics, and religion), irrelevant daydreams, imagining music (2014: 111, 113, 124).

The 'thought examples' provide a vivid indication of a typical runner's bodyworld as she inhabits, via her *specific* physicality, a *specific* material environment while performing a set of *specific* actions. It is as such, by limiting variables to *specificities* of embodiment and pushing them to extremes, that endurance running brings out in higher relief elements that exist in other situations, including in aesthetic performance and daily life.

By occupying a place at the crossroads of such different currents, a closer inspection of 'thoughts' adds to our understanding of the performing body, perhaps contrary to what we have been accustomed to expect in soma-inclined accounts of practices like acting and dancing. For example, as a reading of Phillip B. Zarrilli's deployment of the term 'inhabiting' shows, of the six primary principles he identifies in his account of training for 'psychophysical acting', no less than four foreground the mind (or 'thoughts' as understood in sports science and psychology): attunement of body and *mind*, heightened *awareness*, calibrating of primary *focus*, and, precisely, 'inhabiting dual/multiple *consciousness*' (Camilleri 2013d: 40; Zarrilli 2009: 83, emphasis added). 'Mind', 'awareness', 'focus', and 'consciousness' all involve the body, but the role that 'thoughts' play are rarely acknowledged in the twentieth-century 'turn of the body' (Turner 2012), tainted as they are by Cartesian dualism. Furthermore, the status and details of the body–environment interaction illustrated in the 'thought examples' of sports science and psychology provide down-to-earth concrete details when compared to mind-oriented approaches like neuroscience and situated cognition.

Attentional Focus

It is worth going through Brick et al.'s (2014) categories of attentional focus as a perspective on training and performance with the aim of considering aesthetic and athletic processes in the light of each other. Such an exercise defamiliarizes aesthetic practices like acting and dancing, but also sports disciplines. As far as aesthetic situations are concerned, this defamiliarization engages a 'thought' outlook that has been largely avoided in the wake of the shift to the body as a reaction to Cartesian dualism. Conversely, athletic processes are defamiliarized by their consideration from an unusual angle that focuses on 'performance' as expression, presentation, and communication rather than as competition. To facilitate this reciprocally reflective perspective, Zarrilli's conceptualization of 'the actor's four embodied modes of experience' (2004: 657; 2009: 52–8) can be invoked:

(1) the *first* or '*surface*' body of sensorimotor capacities is outward looking and relies on exteroception;
(2) the *second* or '*recessive*', visceral, body of internal organs and processes is inward looking and interoceptive;
(3) the *third* body or '*aesthetic inner bodymind*' developed in psychophysical training sensitizes an outward/inward dialectic of perception;
(4) the *fourth* or '*aesthetic outer body*' is constituted by the actions or tasks in performance and what spectators see.

As evidenced in Brick et al.'s (2014) review, sports science and psychology tend to consider any cognition, including as it relates to sensory and emotional perception like those included in Zarrilli's categorization, as 'thought' and 'thinking'. When we *register* a sensation, we do so mentally, as a form of thought. On their part, body-based accounts of aesthetic performance like Zarrilli's and Simone Forti's refer to sensations, emotions, and related phenomena like visualization, as essentially or primarily corporeal (Breitwieser 2014). The same applies to occurrences that require heightened mental engagement like attention, focus, and concentration that are conceived as *bodily*. For example,

40 *Performer Training for Actors and Athletes*

intentionality and imagination are frequently discussed in the physical (physiological) terms of impulse (Grotowski in Richards 1995: 96; Barba [1993] 1995: 27–8, 161; Lindh 2010: 25). In such body-based appraisals, the word 'thought' is largely reserved for activities and reflections that are more rational and cerebral, less dependent on specialized embodiments such as prompted by somatic technique. Chapter 4 considers sensations, emotions, and their processing in the context of affect, but for now it suffices to draw attention to this fundamental terminological difference that conditions the ways aesthetic and athletic performance is studied.

The quality of attentional focus in Brick et al.'s category of *active self-regulation*, which deals with running technique (e.g. cadence, stride length, relaxing tense muscles, pacing) and race/training strategy (e.g. when/where to speed up, slow down, keep steady, overtake, or be overtaken), can be aligned with Zarrilli's *aesthetic inner bodymind*, which 'engage[s] the physical body and attention (mind) in cultivating and attuning both to subtle levels of experience and awareness' (Zarrilli 2009: 55). Although concentrating on technique during running requires *internal sensory monitoring*, which includes keeping track of elements that Zarrilli associates with the *recessive/visceral body*, such as breathing, muscle sensations, thirst, and any kind of pain that thematizes aspects usually in the background of consciousness, the athlete seeks to *actively* 'regulate their actions, rather than focusing solely on bodily sensations' (Brick et al. 2014: 110).

In a reference to athletic practice, Zarrilli observes that: 'In the midst of an athletic competition athletes may overcome physical pain as they operate at peak performance' (2004: 660, n. 38), thereby 'braiding and intertwining' (Zarrilli 2009: 59) Brick et al.'s (2014) *internal sensory monitoring* with *active self-regulation*. Indeed, the example Zarrilli discusses at some length with regard to the aesthetic inner bodymind concerns 'attentiveness to the breath' (2009: 55), which is part of the visceral body:

> focusing our attention in and on the act of breathing in a particular way, and in relation to the body, provides one means by which to work against the recessive disappearance of the breath [that characterizes our daily experience of breathing, i.e. we hardly pay attention to it] in order to cultivate the breath and our inner awareness toward a heightened, ecstatic state of engagement in a particular practice and/or in relation to the world.
>
> (2009: 56)

Zarrilli's turn of phrase, 'focusing our attention', converges neatly with Brick et al.'s (2014) 'attentional focus'. Likewise, Zarrilli's emphasis on 'long-term,

Bodyworld Cognitions 41

in-depth engagement' required for the 'subtle level' of awareness in the aesthetic inner bodymind (2009: 55) compares well with the effective 'predominantly associative, task-relevant focus' of elite athletes (Brick et al. 2014: 116). However, is there a difference deeper than a terminological one between, on the one hand, Zarrilli's 'attending to' and visualization ('following with [the] inner eye the breath as it travels in and down along the spine'; 2009: 56) and, on the other hand, Brick et al.'s (2014) 'thinking' or 'cognitions' when it comes to attentional focus? As debated in the following section, the answer might relate not so much to the cognitive processes involved, embodied as they both are, but to their respective *application* in aesthetic and athletic performance.

Movement Aesthetic and Economy

Although the adjective 'aesthetic' in Zarrilli's *aesthetic inner bodymind* is not used in the conventional sense that refers to the stylistic choices and principles pertaining to the organization of presentation, it provides a clue to a fundamental difference with sports. The explanation Zarrilli offers for 'aesthetic' in the context of the 'inner bodymind' is at best implicative about the elusive quality he evokes:

> This process of cultivation and attunement is *aesthetic* in that it is non-ordinary, takes place over time, and allows for a shift in one's experience of the body and mind aspects from their gross separation, marked by the body's constant disappearance, to a much subtler, dialectical engagement of body-in-mind and mind-in-body. It is, therefore, marked as *aesthetic* since *experience is gradually refined to ever-subtler levels of awareness*, and inner since this mode of experience begins with an explanation from within as the awareness learns to explore the body.
>
> (2004: 661, 2009: 55, emphasis added)

The etymology of 'aesthetic' from the Ancient Greek *aisthetikos*, 'of or relating to sense perception', suggests that an aesthetic experience is one that fully engages the senses. In Zarrilli, the reference is bound to a process that refines – and therefore *re-organizes* – one's awareness and capacity for action as distinct from one's daily embodied mode of being/behaving. Except for implied reasons of 'sensorial organization', it is not exactly clear why such refinement is 'aesthetic', especially in Zarrilli's literal deployment of the same word for the fourth body, the *aesthetic outer body*, that is offered on stage for 'the abstractive gaze of the spectator': 'The actor embodies/inhabits these [performance] tasks/actions by dynamically shaping one's energy, attention,

42   *Performer Training for Actors and Athletes*

and awareness to the qualities and constraints of the *aesthetic* form and dramaturgy informing the score' (Zarrilli 2009: 58, emphasis added).

One possible clue to the 'aesthetic' connection between Zarrilli's 'inner bodymind' and 'outer body' emerges in the light of a distinction he seeks to update in phenomenological terms: Eugenio Barba's *pre-expressive* and *expressive* levels of behaviour. For Barba, the pre-expressive in the work of actors and dancers marks 'the elementary level of organization' that is manifested 'transculturally' in 'certain physiological factors [like] weight, balance, the use of the spinal column and the eyes' and 'upon which different genres, styles, roles and personal or collective traditions are all based' ([1993] 1995: 9). Leaving to one side the critique of essentialism often levelled at the pre-expressive (that behaviour is always already 'expressive' and therefore socio-culturally significant, so we are never in a place Barba denotes by '*before* any message is transmitted'), the emphasis on 'recurring principles' implies a capacity for application/training that demands aesthetic filtering ([1993] 1995: 9, emphasis in the original). The expressive level, then, constitutes the specific stylistic choices and cultural inflections that Zarrilli denotes by the aesthetic outer body. According to Barba, pre-expressive scenic behaviour is developed via the '*extra-daily* use of the *body-mind*' techniques ([1993] 1995: 9, emphasis added), which resonates with Zarrilli's 'realm of *extra-daily* perception and experience associated with [...] psychophysical practices or training regimes' that cultivate the aesthetic inner bodymind (2009: 55). From this perspective, the major difference between the aesthetic inner bodymind of theatre/dance performers that I am aligning with the active self-regulation of runners and other athletes involves the question of *expressivity*.

Athletic activity, including running but excluding hybrid forms such as synchronized swimming that combine athleticism with dance aesthetics, is not primarily concerned with expressivity or how an action looks, but with how it *optimally performs*. What 'elegance', 'beauty', or even 'meaning' there is in certain forms or individual styles of athletic behaviour is not driven by aesthetic considerations but perceived by the particular sensibilities of observers. Where it exists, such corporeal 'elegance' is, in most cases, a by-product of what is called 'movement economy'. Although different sports disciplines have specialized versions of it – such as the 'running economy' of runners – *movement economy* refers to goal-directed efficacy. As sports scientist Gabriele Wulf explains in the context of athletic behaviour: 'Skilled performance is characterized by high levels of movement effectiveness and efficiency [...]. That is, a high skill level is associated with accuracy, consistency, and reliability in achieving the movement goal (i.e., effectiveness), as well as fluent and economical movement executions and

Bodyworld Cognitions

automaticity, as evidenced by the investment of relatively little physical and mental effort (i.e., efficiency)' (Wulf 2013: 78).

More succinctly, a 'movement pattern is considered more efficient or economical if the same movement outcome is achieved with less energy expended' (Wulf 2013: 84). This, rather than aesthetics, is what principally concerns athletes. The appraisal of movement economy in elite sports is a methodological science in its own right, overlapping with diagnostic medical technology to measure (and therefore *foreground*) aspects that Zarrilli would classify as 'recessive', including 'muscular (electromyographic or EMG) activity, oxygen consumption, and heart rate' as well as 'maximum force production, movement speed, or endurance' (Wulf 2013: 84). In the specific context of long-distance running and its optimal movement economy:

> Physiological factors related to prolonged endurance performance (e.g., marathon running) include the maximal amount of oxygen that can be utilized (VO_{2max}), lactate threshold (i.e., the intensity at which blood lactate first rises above baseline levels) and movement economy [...]. Running economy (RE) can be defined as the steady-state volume of oxygen consumed (VO_2) during a submaximal running intensity [...] and can explain differences in performance between athletes otherwise matched in terms [of] VO_{2max} and lactate threshold [...].
>
> (Brick et al. 2018: 20)

The insight provided by such data serves to shape an athlete's training and competition practice, precisely with the intention of maximizing and potentially improving their capacity for an optimal movement economy.

As distinct from aesthetic performance, therefore, which by its nature includes the aesthetic gaze and affective response of viewers, athletic sports is concerned with how movement looks only in so far as it efficiently *performs* to its maximal potential. As such, viewed for defamiliarization purposes from a very specific angle that pushes the point to an extreme, athletic performance is constituted of pure movement. 'Pure' in being autotelic, in and of itself, without the additional variables and presentational considerations that necessarily inform aesthetic performance. From the same extreme (and narrow) angle, the 'autotelic purity' of athletic movement epitomizes, in the abstract, Stanislavski's maxim of 'work on oneself' (2008: xv) but without any ulterior motives to express or represent anything beyond human motion. Moreover, in 'meaning' precisely what the body 'does', athletic movement also recalls Artaud's 'theatre of unalienated signs' with its 'visceral and intellectual presence' (Fortier 2016: 55): 'intellectual' precisely because it is *viscerally* so, where the 'objects, the props, even the scenery which will appear on the stage

44   *Performer Training for Actors and Athletes*

will have to be *understood* in an immediate sense, without transposition; they will have to be taken not for what they represent but for what they really are' (Artaud cited in Fortier 2016: 55, emphasis added).

Outward Monitoring

In addition to *internal sensory monitoring* and *active self-regulation*, another related category in Brick et al.'s (2014) model concerns *outward monitoring*, i.e. the perception of events external to the athlete's body. This comprises of environmental factors that pertain to the route and to the race or training session itself (e.g. distance information and water stations). Brick at al. include 'other competitors' as a 'thought example' of this attentional focus while categorizing 'non-competitive runners' as *involuntary distractive*, thereby underlining that 'outward monitoring' involves an evaluation of those external conditions that can impact the athlete's performance to reach her objectives. Brick et al. (2014) also indicate split times as external monitoring, referring to the time taken to complete specific distances (e.g. per kilometre/mile or fractions thereof). Although such information may be available via screens or landmarks during race days or in equipped training environments, the ubiquitous use of personal smart devices (usually watches) makes this data readily and constantly accessible to athletes, especially for the long distances of endurance running but also, literally, for every second of their life (as long as it is strapped around their wrists).

The use of such tracking equipment foregrounds the potential role played by technology vis-à-vis perception, attentional focus, and the impact on performance. In this regard, consider the testimony I provide in *Performer Training Reconfigured* about wearable tracking devices:

> [S]uch apps record my physical performance during running, walking, or cycling in terms of speed, pace, elevation, and distance covered. […] [This technology] makes explicit […] aspects that were previously part of my implicit psychophysical awareness. More significantly from a post-psychophysical perspective, it has become an integral (and therefore *incorporated*) part of my bodymind, of my *embodied consciousness* […] whenever I go running, walking, or cycling with or *without* the app. […] [M]y embodied consciousness of, say, running is now not only attuned to the temperature, the sights and sounds of the surroundings, other people and objects around, and to my psychosomatic performance (e.g. intake of breath, any aches or tensed muscles). My bodymind awareness

Bodyworld Cognitions

is now also informed (*constituted*) by the data that has become available to me. [...] My experience of using the technology has fine-tuned (*trained*) my perception to sense/understand my bodily activity, also drawing attention to environmental factors like heat and wind that affect my performance. [...] I feel an added and assimilated dimension to my exteroception and proprioception. This new awareness I take with me in the theatre studio and forms part of what I call my post-psychophysical bodyworld.

(Camilleri 2019: 76–7, emphasis in the original)

From this perspective, a prolonged and in-depth engagement with such tracking technology *informs* and *forms* one's perception, including the awareness and status of one's feelings, as discussed in Part II. If the 'chiasmatic body' that combines Zarrilli's four embodied modes of experience describes the psychophysical bodymind of actors (2009: 59–60), the overlapping relations between internal sensory monitoring, active self-regulation, and outward monitoring exemplify the post-psychophysical concept of bodyworld. I return to what gets transferred to a theatre scenario later in the chapter, in the meantime I elaborate on my bodyworld as expanded through running praxis.

Four years down the line, I can still vouch for the situation described above in *Performer Training Reconfigured* (2019). If anything, my 'running bodyworld' has been further refined on three principal counts. First, since writing that account, instead of an app on my mobile phone, I have been using a sports watch and a heart monitor that provide a wider, more continuous and accurate range of data, thus extending the perceptual 'fine-tuning' of my activity. Second, I have transitioned from short distances (less than 10 km) to marathon running, which has necessarily entailed a stronger commitment and a more systematic approach to training – 'necessarily' because, as I have learnt, one does not simply run long distances without the requisite physical and mental resilience that is developed over time with sustained preparation. Third, researching for this book involved reading extensively about athletes as well as sports science and sports psychology, thus opening my knowledge–awareness to the intricacies of athletics and athletic bodies. Owing to this three-pronged 'refinement' that impacted the 'chiasmatic' affective–practical–reflective capacities of my 'embodied modes of experience', my 'aesthetic inner bodymind' has sensitized and 'attuned' my ability for active self-regulation during running (Zarrilli 2009: 50–9). The following section exemplifies concrete instances of this refinement.

Running Bodyworld

Endurance and fitness expert Alex Hutchinson considers the flip side of tracking devices when he argues that 'technological enhancements like running with a GPS watch "slacken the bond between perception and action" [...] [because] you're inserting an extra cognitive step that relies on an imperfect external estimate of how you should be feeling, rather than on the feeling itself' (2018: 259). Such 'slackening' is a real possibility if one depends *entirely* on this data and over-rules the 'data' from one's internal monitoring when deciding whether to speed up, slow down, or maintain the current pace. As illustrated below, the key is to strike a balance between disparate sources of information. Even if the technological data may not be 'perfect' there is always the filter of one's *bodyworld experience* that calibrates *one's relationship with that data*, that is, *what one does with it* as informed by the accumulated experience of 'feeling' (see Chapter 4); hence the benefit of extending one's perception sources like the internal and external ones in Brick et al.'s (2014) model.

An example of *active self-regulation* that necessarily involves the effort sensations of *internal monitoring* and the split times (amongst others) of *outward monitoring* concerns certain aspects of running/movement economy. In my case, prior to being made explicit through data tracking, knowledge of these aspects was recessive, or at best vaguely intuitive. Stride length, cadence (measured in 'spm', steps per minute), vertical oscillation (the extent one rises and falls), horizontal oscillation (the extent one sways), and ground contact time (or GCT per split), all describe different features of one's movement. An effective running economy generally entails a higher cadence count, which in turn is associated with lower vertical oscillation (minimizing energy cost) and shorter ground contact time (maximizing dynamic benefit). Likewise, the reduction of horizontal oscillation for a symmetrical balance between left and right foot ground contact time is generally indicative of efficient movement: 'Many runners report that GCT balance tends to deviate farther from 50/50 when they run up or down hills, when they do speed work or when they are fatigued [or injured]' (Garmin 2022). The experience of what I previously *felt*, *perceived*, and therefore also *thought of*, simpl(isticall) y as 'running', as *a single activity*, has now been refined into a complex fusion of reciprocally informing dimensions, or *acts*, of the same phenomenon. Consequently, the awareness of *what* I am doing has been enriched, in the process also enabling me to enhance the performance of *how* I run.

In my case, therefore, an increasingly 'subtler' (in Zarrilli's sense) and more 'knowledgeable' (in Robin Nelson's understanding of reflective '*know what*' and embodied '*know how*'; 2013: 37) running performance

Bodyworld Cognitions

has been accompanied by an improved ability to self-regulate aspects that were previously beyond my aesthetic inner bodymind. Looking back, I can recognize a similar approach that I have refined during my decades-long physical theatre practice, i.e. to break down a task like 'running' into smaller components to enable a focus on specifics such as stride length, cadence, and oscillation. This allows each component to be trained separately as a self-sufficient unit in its own terms before then bringing everything together again during running practice. The process is reminiscent of Grotowski's plastique exercises, where the practitioner rotates different parts of the body (wrists, elbows, shoulders, head, sternum, spine, centre, knees, feet, etc.), first in isolation and then in different combinations, until the entire body is alive – *pulsating* – with the same impulse (see also Chapter 6).

As an example of this de/re-constructive approach, I sought to increase my stride length via yoga positions that involve leg stretches, which I then complemented with 'stride runs' before a race or time trial. Eventually, I settled on twice-weekly yoga sessions to also address recovery issues and minimize injury risk as well as enhance attentional focus. To improve the muscular resilience of my legs, I added twice-weekly weights sessions in my training where I also included torso work to strengthen core and thus improve power for speed. This work was reinforced by regular hill running (repeated runs up and down a hill). Contrary to what I had assumed, muscular capacity rather than stretch flexibility, and therefore weights rather than yoga, is more beneficial for speed and endurance practice; muscular stretching is important for injury prevention and recovery. Another illustration of the cross-training engendered by my 'awakened' (Zarrilli 2009: 57) running bodyworld, involved cycling that, apart from overall conditioning, was directed at optimizing cadence (steps per minute).

My training for aesthetic performance also contributed to specific areas of my running economy. Regarding vertical oscillation, I deployed my awareness from physical theatre exercises (including an adaptation of the horse-riding stance from martial arts) to maintain a steady centre of gravity for better core control to minimize unnecessary energy expenditure. Likewise from my theatre practice, including as inspired by Zarrilli's account, by paying attention to breathing patterns and breath quality, I endeavoured to regulate oxygen intake (and therefore my VO_2 rate) as well as relax unnecessary tension (to further save on energy cost) and foster attentional focus. Moreover, awareness of body posture techniques that are frequently applied or adapted for aesthetic performance, like Alexander Technique and Feldenkrais, provided me with the know-how and know-that to limit horizontal oscillation. This last point brings me back to the question of *expressivity* in aesthetic and athletic performers.

Rehabilitative and exercise therapy practices like Alexander Technique and Feldenkrais were not originally developed for aesthetic purposes but as corrective techniques aimed at musculoskeletal, movement, and even psychological issues. Such techniques, therefore, address and adjust what can be referred to as a body's 'infrastructural economy' that is then applied in different contexts, including in aesthetic performance (see Worth 2015). From a similar viewpoint, the movement economy of athletes can be considered in aesthetic terms. Although the primary objective of improving one's running economy is to produce more effective and efficient movement, the 'work on oneself' entailed by cadence, vertical/horizontal oscillation, GCT, breathing, and so on can result in body configurations and movement patterns that adhere to or recall culturally specific standards or readings of 'elegance' and 'beauty'. As already observed in the frame of 'autotelic purity', such 'elegance' and 'beauty' does not *express* or *signify* anything beyond the movement *itself*, whether it is running, throwing a discus, jumping, or hitting a target. In an aesthetic context like that of a performance, an installation event, or even a painting or a sculpture, the act of running or kicking a football may come to represent, and thus *mean*, 'love', 'hate', 'divinity', 'grace', 'punishment', or whatever, which in itself reveals something not only about the associative capacity of the human mind but also about human movement: that what we read as *expressive* and *aesthetic* in theatre or dance is not inherent in the movement or body but ascribed, attributed, and allocated. Maybe Barba was on the right track, after all, with his problematically *pre-expressive* 'recurring principles' that become expressively significant with specific embodiments ([1993] 1995: 9, 14–34). For what makes something expressive is not inherent but contextual, including the configurations and organization associated with aesthetics. The overlaps and contrasts between the economy and aesthetic of movement are further discussed in Chapter 6.

Distraction

The fourth quality of attentional focus that Brick et al. (2014) classify for endurance activity is sub-divided into *active distraction* and *involuntary distraction*. As the word implies, 'distraction' concerns anything that takes one's attention away from the task at hand, whether it is during the act of running or performing on stage, or even a case of daydreaming in daily life. As such it is often viewed in a negative light that marks a split between the doing body and the thinking mind.

Habitual behaviour is one instance of distracted attention that enacts such a body/mind split. Zarrilli deems habits 'the stupidest thing' because

Bodyworld Cognitions   49

they do 'no good whatsoever' (in Creely 2010: 217), while voice coach Patsy Rodenburg sees them as 'debilitating' (1992: 27). However, the issue is more complex and nuanced than a categorical appraisal of the phenomenon implies. There may be a fine line, with overlapping dimensions, between the 'not-thinking', 'mindlessness', and indeed *distraction* of habitual movement, on the one hand, and the automatic quality of virtuosic performance on the other hand (Camilleri 2018a: 37, 41, 48–9; Camilleri 2019: 159–63). For present purposes, to focus on a specific aspect of training practice, a cue can be taken from Roberta Carreri, an actor who already had forty years' professional experience with Barba's Odin Teatret when she wrote that:

> With daily repetition we learn to work so well with a principle that our body risks engaging what I call the 'automatic pilot'. The mind thinks of something else while the body repeats, for the umpteenth time, a fixed sequence of actions. Instead of reinvigorating us, this split between the mind and the body generates exhaustion. If it happens for many days in succession, it means that it is time to introduce objects or explore new principles in the training.
>
> (Carreri 2014: 61)

It is hard to think of an activity that better epitomizes the 'repetition of a fixed sequence of actions' than long-distance running. And yet, studies from sports science paint an ambivalent picture when it comes to the connection between 'exhaustion' and distraction. In Brick et al.'s review of 112 studies that involve attentional focus in endurance performance, the majority 'that have imposed *active distraction* techniques [...] have indicated either reduced or relatively unaffected effort perceptions during activity' (2014: 112). Likewise with *involuntary distraction*, which has been shown 'to increase enjoyment and reduce boredom [...], to reduce arousal or frustration [...], and to elevate positive moods' (2014: 112). If anything, then, in splitting mind and body, distraction shifts the athlete's attention away from effort perception, and therefore from the experience of exhaustion.

Although in the context of her preceding chapter entitled 'Dialogue with tiredness' Carreri may have been referring to *creative* exhaustion, her emphasis is on physical exhaustion (2014: 58–60), specifically referring to how jogging with an experienced runner makes the effort more bearable: 'the body feels lighter' (58). Carreri attributes this lightness of being to the production of endorphins by the brain (58). But is this not what also happens when 'the body repeats, for the umpteenth time, a fixed sequence of actions'? From a sports science perspective, as Brick et al.'s 'thought examples' for involuntary distraction show with reference to other runners, whether 'conversing' with them or in a 'non-competitive' role (2014: 113), what enabled Carreri to overcome the challenging effort of running may be related to the same 'automatic pilot' she found exhausting in the theatre studio. It is evident that there are various complex factors to consider other than a reductive presumption that habits-are-bad-for-you (Camilleri 2018a). Such a realization exemplifies the kind of defamiliarized insight that ensues from reading aesthetic and athletic performance in the light of each other.

Other findings in Brick et al.'s (2014) review conform with Carreri's understanding of the 'automatic pilot', including that distractive techniques 'generally reduce pace or intensity when compared with self-regulatory cognitions' (114), which implies that in addition to alienating the practitioner from effort sensations, distraction also chips away at one's capacity to reach maximum potential. Moreover, 'greater distraction/dissociation has also been reported during lower-intensity training activities' (114), which resonates with the tendency of sub-par concentration when executing movement patterns or sequences that have been fully mastered (and therefore are no longer challenging enough) or that otherwise require full (psychophysical) engagement for their execution, as Carreri herself discovered when learning acrobatics:

> Acrobatic exercises were fundamental in the formation of all Odin Teatret actors. In the process of learning them, the body and mind must be one: if one *thinks* of other matters while performing an acrobatic exercise, it is highly probable that one will fall and hurt oneself. That is why I like to say that the floor has been my first Zen master: it awoke me each and every time I lost my concentration.
>
> (2014: 27, emphasis added)

A nuanced appreciation of distraction, then, as prompted by Brick et al.'s (2014) model, goes some way in framing the ambivalent signals that accompany instances of 'not thinking about' or 'not focusing upon' the body's current activity. In Vybarr Cregan-Reid's account of running, active distraction overlaps with what he calls 'soft fascination, which is a sort of meandering, free-form mode of thought' usually but not exclusively prompted by natural environments (2016: 106). Rereading my 2019 description of running from Brick et al.'s perspective, I identify an experiential fusion of *active self-regulation* and *active distraction*, with the key overlap being the 'switched on' (i.e. *active*) status of my attentional focus:

> After an initial period of getting accustomed to it (of *training*), the [tracking app] technology has receded to the background of my

Bodyworld Cognitions

consciousness as I run, leap, swerve around obstacles and potholes, cross roads with two-way traffic, prepare for uphill stretches, keep a check on momentum-induced over-exertion during downhill stretches, and so on.

(Camilleri 2019: 77, emphasis in the original)

Preparing for uphill and downhill runs entails *active self-regulation*. Avoiding obstacles, potholes, and traffic falls under the *active distraction* category of 'attention-demanding environment (e.g. urban street)' (Brick et al. 2014: 113). Regarding the latter, although I may not have been focused on aspects of embodiment while running (e.g. on breathing, perspiration, pacing, cadence), I was *not unfocused*, i.e. my attention was not simply drifting (e.g. daydreaming) or *involuntarily distracted*, say, by 'unimportant scenery', but engaged elsewhere. Brick et al.'s (2014) model thus offers a qualified and subtle understanding of distraction.

Being distracted in an *active* way also means being distracted from the perception of effort, which in turn has the potential of enhancing one's performance. Indeed, I am often surprised by the improved pace I always seem to register – without a noticeable change in effort – when I leave the potholes and traffic behind me. Of course, such obstacles occur occasionally or in exceptional circumstances in a run (depending on the route and the event). However, the 'occasionality' of this distraction does not disprove the point. On the contrary, it indicates an existing (inherent or nurtured) capacity. Similar to the discussion in Chapter 5 about the potentially positive effect of periodic or occasional smiling on effort perception and movement economy (Brick et al. 2018: 26), periodic distraction (e.g. as prompted by attention-demanding environments) could be useful and as such deployed strategically.

Automatic Pilot and Exhaustion

The phenomenon of distracted-yet-effective performance can be aligned with 'sensorimotor exigencies', which refer to the transferability of behavioural elements from a specific context to other situations. For example, 'the capacity to move, flowingly and dynamically, and *without thinking* about it, from a backward roll to a headstand [...] can be *engaged* in other everyday life and performance situations' (Camilleri 2019: 198, emphasis in the original). The notion of sensorimotor exigencies builds on J. Kevin O'Regan and Alva Noë's (2001) theory of 'sensorimotor contingencies' that involve the modulated perception of the environment and which operate in the background of consciousness. These contingencies emerge when our attention is directed to our actions due to a change in circumstances (Camilleri 2020b: 22), for example, when suddenly and unpremeditatedly pressing the brake pedal to avoid driving over a cat as it darts across a street. Pertinently to the current discussion, O'Regan and Noë speak of this phenomenon in terms of an 'automatic pilot' (2001: 944), which brings us full circle to Murakami's and Carreri's deployments of the same image.

Similar to Carreri, the autopilot that features in Murakami's ultramarathon is also connected to exhaustion but, unlike Carreri's, is its *consequence* rather than the *cause*: 'I had been transformed [by an overbearing exhaustion] into a being on autopilot, whose sole purpose was to rhythmically swing his arms back and forth, move his legs forward one step at a time. I didn't think about anything. I didn't feel anything' (Murakami 2008: 112). This picture resonates with the shattering of the mental filter that Thomas Richards experienced in that intensive workshop with Grotowski. As noted earlier, Richards danced for 'hours, nonstop. After a certain point, as my physical exhaustion grew, my mind became tired and quiet [...] I felt as if my body started to dance by itself' (Richards 1995: 22–3).

Although expert behaviour is discussed in Chapter 6, it is worth noting a variable that connects Murakami's and Richards' beyond-exhaustion-automaticity: their level of mastery. Even though Murakami was an experienced marathon runner, this was his first ultramarathon. Similarly, although Richards had some experience as an actor, this was his first encounter with Grotowski's work. In other words, both were novices with respect to a task that pushed them to extremes. The case is different with Carreri, who locates her automatic pilot *after* mastering exercises she had been practising for years (Carreri 2014: 61). Carreri's automaticity can be aligned with the triggering of sensorimotor contingencies and exigencies, nurtured in the background of consciousness with repeated practice over a substantial period. Conversely, Murakami's and Richards' experience of a durational and repeated physical activity is located within a much shorter time frame but whose intensity overloaded their cognitive processes *and* physical capacities.

If this hypothesis is correct, how does such an effort-overload enable the physical feats of Murakami's 100 km and Richards' 'body dancing by itself'? On the basis of the information covered in this chapter, it can be proposed that such a somato–cognitive overload leads to a quasi-survival mode that makes maximum use of the resources available, including the adaptation of existing sensorimotor contingencies to 'patch up' deficiencies and cope with the situation. Such maximal deployment comes with a high somatic cost: to accomplish the task it becomes necessary to resort to resources usually reserved for or applied in other purposes, including those of reflective cognition that have been switched off or dimmed in Murakami's and Richards' cases. Such a hypothesis goes some way in contextualizing the suspended or side-tracked cognitive processing, the *'distraction'*, that Murakami and Richards experience through exhaustion; it possibly even tells us something about the meta-/physical 'void' Murakami aspires to when he runs.

The perspective that sports science affords aesthetic performance in this particular instance leads us to review both Richards' novice and Carreri's master experiences as modes of distraction that can be engaged in different ways and at various stages of a practitioner's training. Defamiliarized and modulated in this way, distraction as brought about by intense physical engagement and exhaustion shifts one's attentional capacities on to the performing body, *automatizing the embodiment* at the expense of other more reflective processes of cognition. In its initial phases, when the practitioner is still assimilating the task-learning, such a shift serves to unlock some properties and abilities that, once unlocked, become progressively easier to access without resorting to extreme effort and exhaustion. After all, this is also what happens in daily life when mastering a skill like swimming or riding a bicycle: it takes substantial effort, concentration, and application to acquire but once learnt, you *know* it and cannot 'unknow' or 'unlearn' it unless you experience an injury or a debilitating condition.

Reframed in the light of Brick et al.'s (2014) distinction between active and involuntary distraction, then, the mind/body split that Carreri ascribes to her behavioural automatic pilot becomes not so much a clear-cut attentional deficiency to be avoided at all cost, but a capacity that can be *strategically* engaged to achieve certain objectives in performance, hence the 'attention-demanding tasks (e.g. puzzles)' Brick at al. include as a 'thought example' in endurance activity (2014: 113). Although puzzles and calculations may not be appropriate for aesthetic practitioners *during* performance, Brick et al. provide instances of other 'attention-demanding tasks' that can realistically feature in such situations, like 'rhythmically repeating a phrase' or 'repeating the word "down" on every stride' (114) to remain engaged *through* distraction. This reminds me of a pulse I repeat in my head ('tak tak tak tak tak') in certain instances in training and performing when I am 'doing nothing' or 'going slow' but want to remain psychophysically vigilant. Such 'strategic' uses of distraction or quasi-distraction mark a quality of attentional focus in its own right, albeit not a direct concentration on what the body is doing but one that overlaps with the purposes of active self-regulation. Chapter 2 considers other instances of focus shifts and their implications for optimal performance.

What I Take With Me

In my 2019 account of running with a tracking app, I refer to 'an added and assimilated dimension to my exteroception and proprioception' that 'I take with me in the theatre studio'. This 'new awareness':

> acts upon me in a comparable way that Feldenkrais or Alexander techniques do when enhancing my body awareness in space/posture and time/movement. Just as Feldenkrais, Alexander, and yoga are not 'performer trainings' per se but have been adopted and applied accordingly to performing situations, similarly with the 'new awareness' made available through mobile [phone] technology, which enables the calibration of my body-in-the-world, especially the somatic dimension that involves the efficient generation and maintenance of energy/effort in movement and voice.
>
> (Camilleri 2019: 77)

As indicated earlier, the quality of this 'new awareness' has been refined with my development of a long-distance running practice. What I had previously identified in general terms as 'the psychosomatic aspects' of running, such as the 'flexibility, stamina, and breath control' that were transferred to my studio work (2019: 77), have evolved into more specific and sophisticated knowledge (as embodied *know how* and reflective *know that*). This enhanced knowledge revolves around motion and endurance, particularly with reference to breathing and muscular demands as influenced by cadence, pacing, balance (in ascending/uphill, descending/downhill, and level terrains), as well as the constant corporeal adjustments required by these and other elements. Importantly, my understanding and application of focus has been transformed, not only *during* running as exemplified in this chapter by Brick et al.'s (2014) model of embodied and environmental awareness, but perhaps more so when it comes to *pre*-performance *preparation*.

In my case, preparing for a long run entails not only the appropriate physical organization associated with fitness, rest/recovery, and nutrition, but also a specific attitude as discussed in more detail in Chapter 2 in the context of the mind-over-muscle debate. This attitude, which I consider as a kind of mental 'positioning', 'setting', or 'modality', is ever-present during a weeks-long marathon programme and shifts between background and foreground consciousness according to the proximity of the weekly long run in question. Similar to the skill-learning process discussed in the previous section, in the lead-up to my first marathon, this kind of pre-performance

Bodyworld Cognitions

'mental positioning' was almost semi-permanently in the foreground, no doubt because I was facing unknown territory with every long run, progressing from 21 km to 24 km, 27 km to 30 km, 35 km to 37 km, and finally 42.2 km.

A vital aspect of this 'mental positioning' included visualization of the route, a form of visual *and embodied* rehearsal of the conditions I expected to encounter along the way regarding the road, climate, time of day, and so on but also, crucially, my anticipated psycho/physical states (sensorial and emotional feelings) at various locations and moments, especially in the 'unknown' stretches towards the end. This must have served as a coping mechanism for the upcoming challenge. Theatre actor and teacher Neal Utterback taps specifically into this kind of rehearsed 'mental imagery' from sports psychology as a technique for student-actors to imaginatively anticipate and develop 'protocols' to resolve potential issues when performing in front of an audience (Utterback 2016: 84). Indeed, sports writer and coach Matt Fitzgerald speaks of 'a highly developed overall coping capacity in endurance sports' in terms of *mental fitness* that needs to be nurtured (2016: 12).

With experience, this kind of preparation (or *training*), which marks a form of *focus*, stayed with me but no longer occupying centre stage for days before a run. I learnt to modulate it, heightening it in the preceding 24 hours in a way that I felt *ready* by the time I took the first steps in the run. The enhanced and subtle awareness developed in the durational course of and the depth of engagement with this practice has been assimilated within my aesthetic inner bodymind. And this 'mental positioning' or 'mental fitness' is precisely what I now take with me into the theatre studio.

Zarrilli associates the aesthetic inner bodymind with 'long-term, in-depth engagement in certain psychophysical practices or training regimes – yoga, the martial arts, *butoh*, acting/performing per se, or similar forms of embodied practice which engage the physical body and attention (mind) in cultivating and attuning both to subtle levels of experience and awareness' (Zarrilli 2009: 55). Along with elements from disciplines like yoga, acrobatics, dance, and martial arts that through the years I have learnt in order to supplement and improve my physical training for performance and practical teaching purposes, I can now include long-distance running. Apart from physical dexterity (especially now that mine is no longer a young body), what running has given me better or more than other disciplines is a concrete, even pragmatic, appreciation of the performing body. Long-distance running has provided me with a meditational practice in motion, teaching me patience and control, when to hold back, keep steady, and surge forward, in the process shaping and modulating my aesthetic inner bodymind. If the floor was Roberta Carreri's professed 'first Zen master' when she was learning acrobatics, I have found the road an excellent bodyworld teacher because on a long run there are no half measures in the relationship with your own self and the world around: you either run the distance or you fall short. And to do that, you prepare.

2

Mind Your Body:
Attentional Focus in Performance

When Haruki Murakami went past the three-quarter mark during his epic 100 km ultramarathon (see Chapter 1), his legs ceased to protest (Murakami 2008: 112). The 'autopilot' that left him bereft of thought and feeling kicked in, almost literally *kicking* him forward, to such an extent that he might have continued running beyond the finishing line (113). His muscles had the capacity to drive him forward, even beyond the point he *thought* and *felt* he could not run any longer. From the perspective of the 3As of bodyworld (see Introduction), the specific *affordances* of Murakami's muscles enabled him to complete the task. He hints at such a capacity while connecting it to body/mind and nature/nurture relationalities:

> [Mine are] the kind of muscles you need for long distances. [...] I feel that this type of muscle is connected to the way my mind works. What I mean is, a person's mind is controlled by his body, right? Or is it the opposite – the way your mind works influences the structure of the body? Or do the body and mind closely influence each other and act on each other? What I do know is that people have certain inborn tendencies [...]. Tendencies can be adjusted, to a degree, but their essence can never be changed.
>
> (Murakami 2008: 84)

Murakami's raw articulation, without 'any technical details' from science or elite practice but sourced from personal experience (2008: 84), is precisely the reason he is evoked here, for he lays bare, in stark terms, central questions that concern this book: the connections between body, mind, and world, and the extent to which these are trainable for aesthetic and athletic purposes.

Regarding the question of 'certain inborn tendencies', although Murakami's muscles eventually demonstrated that they could take a 100 km ultramarathon, they still needed the preparation that came with his daily runs and regular marathons. Thus, although not everyone has the *ability* to be an Olympic medallist, or an exceptional aesthetic performer for that

58   *Performer Training for Actors and Athletes*

matter, everyone – irrespective of their body shape and condition – has the *capacity* to train and improve their 'tendencies'. As such, the question of 'inborn tendencies' and 'their essence' can be reformulated in bodyworld terms of assemblages, affordances, and actants relating to a combination of geographical, environmental, socio-cultural, technique, and individual factors. A specific illustration of such factors is the 'altitude, training, culture, and runners' determination' (Pasley 2019) that epitomize the best runners in the world today: Kenyans and Ethiopians from the Rift Valley area (Fitzgerald 2016: 157).

The present chapter continues from the preceding one in re-evaluating the role played by the embodied mind in somatic practices. It specifically explores matters relating to attentional focus, the 'mind–muscle connection', and behavioural automaticity, thus supplying some of the 'technical details' missing in Murakami's account. While the 'mind–muscle connection' is juxtaposed with psychophysicality in aesthetic processes with the aim of shedding light on both practices, automaticity is considered with reference to 'choke' and flow experiences. The issue of tendencies is addressed more broadly from the perspective of affordances in the Introduction and of affect in Chapter 4.

Internal/External Focus and the Mind–Muscle Connection

Sports scientist and motor learning specialist Gabriele Wulf is often linked with the development of a new approach to the study of attentional focus in performing athletes. Just as Chapter 1 considered thinking modalities and strategies as either broadly 'associative' or 'dissociative' to indicate the *monitoring* of physical sensations or their *distraction* in performance, Wulf and various colleagues have examined the phenomena from the perspective of *external* and *internal* focus, with the first study dating to 1998 (Wulf et al. 1998).

It is important to clarify at the outset that 'attentional focus' does not equate to 'visual focus' but refers to the performer's concentration. Wulf specifies that in such instances 'visual information is typically kept constant […] by asking participants to look straight ahead' (Wulf 2013: 79). In this model, an *external focus* directs the performer's attention to the movement effect, or to an implement deployed during movement, or to the environment more widely. With *internal focus*, the thought process of the individual rests on a specific movement of muscle or the body. In a wide-ranging review of more

Attentional Focus in Performance 59

than 100 studies published over fifteen years, Wulf found overwhelming evidence that, relative to internal focus, external attention 'enhances motor performance and learning' across 'different types of tasks, skill levels, and age groups', specifically with regard to '*movement effectiveness*, such as balance or accuracy, and *movement efficiency*, as measured by muscular activity, maximum force production, speed, or endurance' (2013: 77, 78, emphasis in the original).

From an aesthetic performance outlook, the internal/external modality appears at first glance to be reminiscent of psychophysicality's distinction between inner and outer action (Camilleri 2013d). Outer action refers to the shape or design – even style – of a physical/vocal score, exercise, or choreography. Inner action indicates a performer's organic engagement of capacities like intentionality, emotions, memories, and imagination in the execution of movement. Phillip Zarrilli writes about awakening and activating 'inner energy' to attune body and mind together (2009: 83), which consequently results in 'constantly felt inner movement' (2020: 28). Theoretically and practically speaking, an outer action of a performance score or training exercise can be completed while thinking about something else. From a psychophysical perspective, such an occurrence marks a split between body and mind that is generally considered deficient like the habitual, mechanized, and distracted behaviour discussed in Chapter 1. The current chapter examines a more nuanced appraisal of intentional distraction in sports that is sometimes used to enhance athletes' performance.

According to Zarrilli, the capacities of inner action can be cultivated through techniques like the sensitization of the 'inner eye', which is a specific and more encompassing form of visualization:

when we *actively* utilize our 'inner eye' ('mind's eye' or active imagination) *we are no longer bound by the constraints of the visual field of sight per se.* Visualization as a way of working with the active imagination can be described as a voluntary psychophysical act in which one engages and then sustains one's attention (and the ancillary awareness that arises from attending to) over time [...].
(Zarrilli 2020: 123, emphasis in the original)

The expanded visualization of Zarrilli's 'inner eye' or 'active imagination' chimes with the 'potential multisensory nature of the imagery experience' explored by sports psychologists in the debate of 'whether imagery is conceptualized as a *quasi-perceptual phenomenological experience* or as a *mental representation*' (MacIntyre et al. 2019: 628, emphasis in the original). In Zarrilli's case, it is helpful to conceive of the 'inner eye' within the frame

60   *Performer Training for Actors and Athletes*

of 'quasi-perceptual phenomenological experience'. This is evidenced by the detailed description he provides of 'following' (i.e. visualizing) the movement of one's breath as it travels *feelingly* down to and up from below the navel area (2009: 25–6; 2020: 124–5). Amongst other goals, this meditational breath-control exercise serves to synchronize the practitioner's 'external and inner eyes', locating them in the lower abdomen (2020: 125).

From Wulf's angle, Zarrilli's 'inner eye' approximates a classic case of internal focus during the act of breathing. Indeed, Zarrilli's expanded understanding of visualization can be aligned with what undoubtedly classifies as internal focus in sports: the mind–muscle connection (Camilleri 2020b: 21). The mind–muscle approach in resistance training (i.e. strength training often associated with the use of weights) entails *imagining contracting* a specific group of muscles whilst *actually flexing them*, e.g. the pectoralis major during a bench press. As such, the 'use of the mind-muscle principle [...] may be considered as a kind of *mental imagery technique* (*but including motor execution* at the same time)' (Calatayud et al. 2017: 1451, emphasis added). An external focus of the same exercise would involve the same 'outer' actions and implements but concentrating on an aspect of the environment, like the barbell in a bench press (Halperin and Vigotsky 2016: 863). Although from a *physical* viewpoint Zarrilli's 'active imagination' for breath control appears relatively static compared to weight training, both practices involve *visualizing* an aspect of the visceral/internal dimension of the body (see Chapter 1), i.e. 'what the tensing and relaxing of specific muscles looks and feels like *while actively doing the action*. Both cases aim to achieve the object of their imagination by the process of enacting it visually and sensorially' (Camilleri 2020b: 21, emphasis in the original).

As already noted, Wulf's extensive research and literature review present 'conclusive' evidence across the board that an external focus is more effective than an internal one when it comes to motor performance and learning (Halperin and Vigotsky 2016: 863). The only exception where 'a control condition was superior to one with an instructed external (and internal) focus' concerned world-class balance acrobats (Wulf 2008): their 'automaticity [...] was disrupted by the additional focus instructions' (Wulf 2013: 96). The issue here is related to a practice that demands highly specialized behaviour whose precision relies on an exceptional degree of automaticity. I return to questions of automaticity in the context of expert performance later in the present chapter and in Chapter 6.

The only dimension where an internal focus is beneficial relative to external attention concerns the mind–muscle connection in resistance training. However, the advantage is not related to motor efficiency, precision, and learning, but to the increase in muscular bulk of hypertrophy (Calatayud

Attentional Focus in Performance 61

et al. 2016; Calatayud et al. 2017). In Wulf's review this is borne out in studies that resulted in lower muscular activity but enhanced movement accuracy when an external focus was applied (Wulf 2013: 84). Brad J. Schoenfeld and Bret Contreras conveniently sum up the internal/external focus debate and its practical implications for different sport disciplines thus:

> Attentional focus should match the goal of the task. Competitive sport athletes should rely heavily on external attentional focus in practice and during games or matches. This includes powerlifters, weightlifters, or strongmen seeking to set a 1RM [one-repetition maximum] or to maximize force or torque production; basketball players or track & field athletes seeking to maximize jump height or distance; runners or rowers seeking to improve economy; and dart throwers, golfers, and pool players seeking maximum accuracy. Alternatively, when attempting to maximize muscle activation, an internal focus of attention would seem to be a better choice. Bodybuilders, physique athletes, and others seeking maximal hypertrophy will conceivably benefit by focusing on the target muscle during an exercise rather than on the outcome or environment.
> (Schoenfeld and Contreras 2016: 28)

In short, external focus is recommended for movement precision, and internal focus for muscular volume. In both instances, the body's performance (and shape) is conditioned by the mind.

Flow Automaticity

Do the sports science findings on internal/external attentional focus have any relevance to aesthetic performance processes, perhaps as they relate to the associative/dissociative cognitive qualities discussed in Chapter 1? Or are we dealing with different psychosomatic realities despite the apparent inner/ outer echoes? It is worth considering such questions with reference to the discussion on mind–body relationalities.

One of the studies in Wulf's review – by Robert A. Duke, Carla Davis Cash, and Sarah E. Allen (2011) – deals with musicians, specifically piano players who were asked to play a sequence of alternating semiquaver notes 'as quickly and evenly as possible [...] under four conditions: with a focus on their finger movements, on the movements of the piano keys, on the hammers, or on the sound of the keyboard' (Wulf 2013: 83). On a transfer test, which assesses motor skills similar to but not the same as the ones practised, it was found that 'a focus on the more distal movement effects

62 *Performer Training for Actors and Athletes*

(sound or hammers) resulted in greater consistency than either focusing on the more proximal effect (keys) or the internal focus (fingers)' (2013: 83; Duke et al. 2011: 48–50). Although these results do not tell us anything specific about seminal aesthetic concerns, such as the *interpretation* of playing those notes (that in turn is bound up with emotional feeling, communicative ability, and lived experience), they do say something about the quality and precision of motor execution. The results suggest an aspect of performance that is not exclusively linked to technical mastery but which overlaps with it, i.e. to its conditions and consequences. Without placing the full weight of the argument on Duke et al.'s study, their findings on the musicians' 'greater consistency' when focusing distally can be taken as a cue to align the phenomenon with the concept of *flow*, precisely to highlight the kind of insight that can be garnered when looking at aesthetic and athletic practices in the light of each other.

Psychologist Mihaly Csikszentmihalyi's research on 'optimal experience' has become synonymous with a conceptualization of 'flow' that marks a highly focused mental state conducive to productivity in various situations (Csikszentmihalyi and Csikszentmihalyi 1988), including in somatic contexts like sports (Jackson and Csikszentmihalyi 1999). In an article on performer process, theatre practitioner and trainer John Britton draws on Csikszentmihalyi's nine descriptors of flow (Csikszentmihalyi 1990; Jackson 1996: 77) to map them against the work of theatre-makers Eugenio Barba, Phillip Zarrilli, Vsevolod Meyerhold, and his own:

[1] There are clear goals at every moment of the activity.
[2] There is immediate [and '*unambiguous*'] feedback to one's actions.
[3] There is a balance between challenges and skills.
[4] There is no worry of failure. [...]
[5] Action and awareness are merged.
[6] Distractions are excluded from consciousness [i.e. 'total *concentration on the task at hand*'].
[7] Self-consciousness disappears.
[8] The sense of time becomes distorted. [...]
[9] The activity becomes autotelic (i.e. an end in itself).
> (Britton 2010: 39; additional text from Jackson 1996: 77, emphasis in the original)

While the first four dimensions involve prerequisite conditions, the rest deal with the phenomenology of the state.

Susan A. Jackson, who co-wrote *Flow in Sports* (1999) with Csikszentmihalyi, provides a clearer articulation of the fourth characteristic listed by Britton. It is of particular relevance to the present discussion about the *effects* of internal and external attentional focus *and their causes* when she describes it as: 'The *paradox of control* [... where] one has a sense of exercising control without trying to be in control during flow' (Jackson 1996: 77, emphasis in the original). Such a contradictory state is recognized by experienced athletes and aesthetic performers who let go of micro-managing their actions (such as occurs in instances of internal focus that monitor the body's performance) when they are in full flow, *feeling* at one with their actions and aspirations. Importantly, Jackson points out that flow is not necessarily the same thing as 'peak performance', even if the two are related: while peak performance denotes 'a standard of accomplishment' that can be verified externally (e.g. by a chronometer), flow designates a feeling and 'psychological state' and as such is subjective (1996: 76).

Csikszentmihalyi provides further insight into the phenomenon of flow when he refers to it as 'an *almost automatic*, effortless, yet *highly focused* state of consciousness' (1996: 110, emphasis added). 'Almost automatic' because this is not a mindless occurrence but, again paradoxically, a form of cognition that *supersedes* – rather than falls short of – conscious thinking, i.e. a specific state of *focused* embodied cognition that replaces rational thought or, for that matter, merely mechanized movement. In an account of music and sports improvisation from the perspective of flow, psychiatrist and neuroscientist Nelson Maldonato and colleagues observe that:

> For an actor, a dancer, or a musician – so absorbed by their action as to be entirely identified with their own task – concentration, automatisms, and imagination build on the real-time flow of action itself (i.e., the intrinsic capability of automated goal-oriented actions to anticipate their own bodily outcomes), rather than on a detached representational schema of the movement to be executed [...].
>
> (Maldonato et al. 2019: 701)

This notion of a sophisticated bodily cognition that transcends schematic patterns resonates strongly with Odin Teatret performer Julia Varley's experience of having 'other thoughts' when 'totally concentrated' and performing a sequence of actions:

> My thoughts are free even if deeply rooted and present in the action. [...] I am present through the precision of the score that I have incorporated not absent in a schematic structure that hides the surroundings from me. The body is intelligent, ready, not mechanical, after it has liberated itself from the difficulty of remembering.
>
> (Varley [1995] 2021: 215, 216)

Varley provides various examples of such 'simultaneous' thoughts, ranging from 'technical observations' about the performance (e.g. light cues), 'practical considerations' that do not concern the performance (e.g. post-show activities), to 'new interpretations of the performance' that emerge when she makes fresh associations about certain details on stage ([1995] 2021: 215).

Although the same or similar thoughts in other situations might serve as a distraction – of the 'involuntary' kind to use Brick et al.'s (2014) classification from Chapter 1 – the highly focused context in which Varley operates presumes both (1) mastery of technique (i.e. ability to execute) and (2) complete assimilation of the performed material. Such conditions generally accompany the full-time engagement of professional practice. Indeed, Varley, an experienced performer and trainer of many decades' standing, calls this a 'state of being' that she ascribes to 'continuous repetition' and 'obsessively detailed' rehearsal work *as well as* performing the piece 'at least thirty times' ([1995] 2021: 216). This picture matches the one painted by sports scientists with regard to automaticity in expert performance by elite athletes (e.g. Jackson 1996: 77; Moran 2012: 87–8; Baker and Farrow 2015; Cappuccio 2019: xx; Cappuccio et al. 2019: 111–13), including by Csikszentmihalyi in his accounts of flow (Jackson and Csikszentmihalyi 1999). Against this background, therefore, automaticity is not the side-effect of a lazy or incomplete process that relies on a bag of tricks. Rather, it is the consequence of a long and intense practice that constantly seeks to enhance one's capacity to push psychosomatic limits.

Maldonato et al. argue that any 'sensorial and cognitive interferences' to such assimilated and automatized processes 'risk reactivating conscious control, compromising the fluidity of the movement and bringing the action back under the control of explicit decision making' (2019: 701). This resonates with findings from the internal/external focus debate, specifically with the *constrained action hypothesis* by Gabriele Wulf, Nancy McNevin, and Charles H. Shea (2001), which states that 'an internal focus induces a conscious type of control, causing individuals to constrain their motor system by interfering with automatic control processes. In contrast, an external focus promotes a more automatic mode of control by utilizing unconscious, fast, and reflexive control processes' (Wulf 2013: 91). Studies indicate connections and overlaps between external focus instructions and various measures of automaticity, including (1) evidence of 'reduced attentional-capacity demands', i.e. less to think about and process during motor execution; (2) 'high-frequency movement adjustments', i.e. more space and capability for action (anticipation) and reaction (response); and (3) 'reduced pre-movement times, representing more efficient motor planning' (Wulf 2013: 91), i.e. enhanced action readiness (see also Chapter 4).

Attentional Focus in Performance   65

Based on corollary research, Wulf and Rebecca Lewthwaite have subsequently proposed that an internal focus possibly acts as a 'self-invoking trigger' that activates self-evaluative and self-regulatory processing and which in turn results in 'a series of ongoing "microchoking" episodes with attempts to right thoughts and bring emotions under control' (Wulf and Lewthwaite 2010: 93, 94). Aidan Moran makes much the same point when he contrasts flow with 'choking':

> First, athletes who choke tend to report that the more deliberately they strive to excel, the worse their performance becomes. Therefore, choking seems to occur, paradoxically, because people try *too* hard to perform well. Second, choking is characterised by an internal focus of attention in which athletes become self-conscious and think too much about the mechanics of their skills.
>
> (Moran 2012: 88, emphasis in the original)

The researchers of the piano-playing exercise relate to such an explanation, arguing that 'participants performed more effectively when they were able to recruit automatized components of long-practised motor behavior by focusing on the effects that their movements produced, rather than focusing on the movements themselves' (Duke et al. 2011: 51). I return to 'choking' and its equivalent in an aesthetic context, 'stage fright', in Chapter 4. In the meantime, it can be deduced from the abundant evidence available that flow and external attention share a high degree of affinity when it comes to automaticity in situations of heightened concentration. The same cannot be said for instances of internal attention like self or execution focus. In this light, therefore, automaticity does not correspond to mindless behaviour but to a shift 'to an unconscious mode of control' in expert performers (Moran 2012: 88; cf. Gray 2015: 74–5), hence Csíkszentmihályi's paradox of control.

Epistemic Actions in Performance

Wulf's review contains a section on possible future studies to address certain limitations in our understanding of attentional focus. She includes three areas that intersect with dimensions of particular interest to aesthetic performers: (1) skills that exclude implements (like 'diving'), (2) skills 'judged by form (e.g., figure skating)', and (3) 'longer-duration serial skills, such as a pole vault or even a gymnastics routine, that involve different sub-routines' (Wulf 2013: 98). Actors, dancers, and performance artists can relate to processes that do not involve any equipment, that are reliant on movement design

66   *Performer Training for Actors and Athletes*

or style for their messaging/appreciation, and that consist of extended and overlapping sequences with various skill combinations of speaking, singing, moving, acting, and dancing, sometimes even while using 'implements' like playing a musical instrument or handling objects or a weapon (e.g. fencing) on stage. The first of these three instances requires some explanation.

Although many aesthetic performers are accustomed to working without any 'implements', they are hardly as materially *divested* (as in the etymological sense of 'undressed') as the example of diving Wulf mentions, and as such are potentially comparable to runners in resorting to clothes, the ground, or environmental landmarks for external focus. Wulf's review includes various studies on running (2013: 87–9) that provide pointers for actors and dancers in this regard, including one that tested 'an external focus (i.e., clawing the floor with the shoes), compared with an internal focus (i.e., moving the legs and feet down and back as quickly as possible) or a control condition (i.e., running as quickly as possible)' (88). In other words, aesthetic performers who do not use any implements operate in conditions (e.g. wearing costumes, inhabiting stage sets, sharing spaces with a public) that make external attentional focus less of an issue than contemplated by Wulf. Indeed, some of the 'simultaneous other thoughts' that occur to Varley during performance include lighting equipment, items of costume (her own and a fellow actor's), and an audience member ([1995] 2021: 215).

Therefore, even when a performer does not use any implements, she is often in the *presence* of materialities that can serve a similar function, which in turn affects her bodyworld and thus her scenic *presence*, hence necessarily involving her attentional engagement. After all, this is what post-psychophysical perspectives afford in acknowledging body–mind–world intra-relationalities (Camilleri 2019: 1–2, 33–4). As a consequence of such 'states of being', insights from the performing arts can contribute a different perspective to the discussion on the internal/external dimensions of attentional focus. To this end, a theatre-oriented reading of 'epistemic actions' (Camilleri 2019: 206–10) can be evoked to tease out implications that can be compared with the attentional dynamics of secondary tasks in sports.

Cognitive scientists David Kirsh and Paul P. Maglio (1994) distinguish between *pragmatic actions* that seek to accomplish a goal as directly as possible (e.g. to pick an apple from a tree) and *epistemic actions* that modify an aspect of the environment to solve a problem or complete a task (e.g. to climb and stand on a chair to extend one's reach to pick an apple from a tree). Epistemic actions are '*external* actions that an agent performs to change his or her own [internal] computational state' to make it 'easier, faster, or more reliable' to achieve the intended objective (1994: 513–14, emphasis in the

Attentional Focus in Performance 67

original). They are often not immediately logical (i.e. pragmatic) in adopting a seemingly roundabout or digressive way of proceeding.

Transposed to aesthetic performance, epistemic actions include memory aids like note-taking after training or rehearsing with a script in hand prior to memorizing it. Preparing the workplace is another type of epistemic actions identified by Kirsh and Maglio, which, in a theatre scenario include setting up props, costumes, and other implements as well any spatial markings on stage. Epistemic actions that are more directly related to the *content* of aesthetic performance concern the research of background material for a character in a psychological realist play or visual inspiration (e.g. from photographs or paintings) for a dance choreography or physical theatre piece. These content-related 'exploratory actions' fall under what Kirsh and Maglio call 'information gathering activities' (1994: 515). Paradoxically, therefore, these additional actional manoeuvres – said to have an epistemic 'function' or 'reach' – are intended to achieve a more economical, efficient, and accurate outcome.

Theatre practitioner and researcher Rebecca Loukes evokes epistemic actions in her consideration of an extended bodymind for performers, i.e. to see whether certain aspects of cognitive processing can be 'extended' to or 'offloaded' on elements of the situating environment (for a comparison with the concept of bodyworld see Camilleri 2019: 208–9). She argues that, due to the various compositional and skill requirements demanded by aesthetic performance, 'we could view the learning of a sequence of movements in yoga, or the creation and assimilation of a physical "score" of actions as a "meta-system" of epistemic actions' (Loukes 2013: 242). Indeed, the purpose of learning skills from a variety of sources not related to theatre (including martial arts, acrobatics, and sports) is 'not pragmatic' in that one does not need to be an acrobat or a martial artist to be an actor. Such skills are pragmatic only if a performance score demands the representation of specific movements, say, for a fight or dance sequence. In the words of Zarrilli, and as discussed in Chapter 1 with reference to sensorimotor exigencies, such practices cultivate a performer's 'aesthetic inner bodymind' (i.e. they sensitize one's awareness while enhancing one's physical capabilities), which constitutes the basis for the 'aesthetic outer bodymind' (the roles and characters) that audiences see on stage.

Loukes proposes other ways the performer's work can be considered epistemically, including viewing the work of Stanislavski on physical actions as 'a method of extending our "epistemic reach"' because using physical actions to develop a character can be arguably viewed as offloading the 'mental' work onto our environment (Loukes 2013: 242). The emphasis on personal experience and imagination in Stanislavski's detailed approach

68   *Performer Training for Actors and Athletes*

conceivably serves an epistemic function when building a character. As Stanislavski scholar Jean Benedetti argues:

> In the method of Physical Action [...] the actor starts by creating, *in his own person*, very often in precise detail, a logical sequence of actions, based on the question, 'What would I do *if* ... ', the 'if' being his intentions within the given circumstances of the play. [...] The actor's total being is therefore engaged from the start. The circumstances and the actions they prompt become, in the process of exploration, a personal reality.
> (Benedetti 2000: 91, emphasis in the original)

In Stanislavski's work, this 'personal reality' is carefully constructed bit by bit (Aquilina 2016: 114–15), illustrating a case of *scaffolded epistemic dynamics* (Camilleri 2019: 208). Similar to Zarrilli's aesthetic inner bodymind, this nurtured 'personal reality' gives shape to and becomes integral to the outer bodymind that audiences see on stage: 'The process of character-creation is not one of self-effacement but of self-transformation whereby one's own life experiences become the experience of the character. A third being is created, a fusion of the character the author wrote and the actor's own personality, the actor/role' (Benedetti 2000: 95). This 'fusion of being' is discussed in the following section but here it serves to underline the apparently non-pragmatic activities that characterize the creation of an onstage persona.

Apart from Stanislavski-based processes of psychological realism that require actors to embody scripted roles, similar permutations apply to the 'action-possibilities' inherent in situations of devised aesthetic composition, which includes collaborative work with other practitioners, whether performers, writers, or designers, as well as working with objects (Camilleri [2020] 2022). Loukes illustrates such 'action-possibilities' through her own personal performance work (2013: 248–52). From this perspective, then, aspects of puppetry, site-specific, and applied performance work are also *scaffolded on* the materiality of objects and sites (Camilleri 2019: 208), thus signalling other examples of 'mental' offloading mechanisms.

Secondary Tasks

Without conflating the epistemic aspects in aesthetic performance with secondary tasks in sports, it is possible to detect resonances in the constitution and quality of attentional focus in both phenomena. Before delving into the connections, it is important to highlight the divergences, including a fundamental ontological one. That is, while aesthetic epistemic actions mark

Attentional Focus in Performance   69

outcome-relevant-if-indirect tasks, i.e. the objective remains the staging of a performance, secondary tasks in sports are predominantly a methodological device, often non-discipline relevant, deployed by researchers with limited applicability beyond the laboratory (Land 2007: 19; Land and Tenenbaum 2007), e.g. counting backwards during the primary task of kicking a ball.

Secondary tasks – also known as 'dual tasks' – are employed to distract attention from a primary task with the aim of triggering expert automatic behaviour that is learnt, mastered, and enhanced during extensive training. This function of secondary tasks links directly with the issues discussed earlier about the self-evaluative and self-regulatory processing associated with choking during internal focus. That is, by engaging in such tasks it is envisaged that the individual's capacity for self-analysis is reduced (and with it the risk of 'paralysis by analysis') to facilitate the flow experience required for peak performance.

Although the research and applied settings of secondary tasks in sports distinguish them from the 'real-life' aesthetic situations targeted by epistemic activity in the performing arts, both phenomena are, in fact, developed in the *laboratory* of practice. The training and rehearsal approaches mentioned above, including Stanislavski's and more recent developments in performance-making, are associated with *research* that 'tests' (explores and develops) various psychophysical and compositional strategies in the studio. This activity is reflected in the terminology of a theatre or dance 'workshop' and 'workshopping' a scene. Indeed, the word 'laboratory' itself is linked with key historical developments in the twentieth century (Schino 2009; Brown 2019) and even features in the name of ensembles like Grotowski's Teatr Laboratorium and Odin Teatret's Nordisk Teaterlaboratorium.

The laboratorial (experimental) quality of both phenomena exposes something that is equally ontological regarding the non-pragmatic processes involved, whether it is the higher actional cost but ultimately performance-effective *indirect* epistemic actions engaged by aesthetic practitioners (i.e. executing scaffolded actions to arrive at the end product), or the equally high processing load of having an additional (secondary) task that is also aimed at an optimal outcome. Despite the extra burdens involved – or rather, *because* of them as studies show – aesthetic and athletic practitioners perform more effectively in sensorimotor *and* phenomenological terms as evidenced respectively by the scientific measurements in sports science (cf. movement economy in Chapter 1) and the experiential assessments of flow (cf. Csikszentmihalyi's work).

In addition to the requisite skill mastery, the efficacy of such strategies is not compromised by the extra computational/cognitive loads but, on the contrary, *facilitated* by a modal shift of attention. As a group of sports

70 *Performer Training for Actors and Athletes*

psychologists and cognitive scientists argue with reference to major empirical studies on choking in sports:

> Self/execution focus impairs the normal course of skillful actions not because it increases the computational burden [cf. 'even secondary tasks that heavily rely on working memory do not significantly affect the sensorimotor performances of the experts'], but because it decomposes the habitual action routines into disconnected segments and clumsy step-by-step procedures, preventing fluid and adaptive on-line control. That is why choking is occasionally characterized as "paralysis by analysis" […].
>
> (Cappuccio et al. 2019: 113)

Although 'automaticity' – and even more so the idea of 'automatized routines' – has connotations of mindless and lifeless behaviour in aesthetic performance, especially in psychophysical approaches that emphasize total presence in the here and now (Camilleri 2018a: 38–41), it does not mean – as already observed – that the agent is *not* focused. As Varley notes from her extensive experience with regard to the 'other thoughts' that may feature in her consciousness when performing:

> The idea that an actress has to be totally present in the action, at one with what she is doing, gives a picture of a body/mind in which thought is indissolubly bound to action; as if I ought not think of anything else. Nevertheless, during a performance, while present in my action and *totally concentrated*, I discover *the simultaneous presence of other thoughts* […].
>
> (Varley [1995] 2021: 215, emphasis added)

She hits on an important point when she insightfully continues:

> I can be *occupied* by different thoughts without these detracting from my presence on stage, but I cannot be *preoccupied* by them. The thoughts must not be at the centre of my attention, nor should they determine the accent of the whole picture. Most importantly, I should not think about the score and thus create a separation within me as an actress […].
>
> (215, emphasis in the original)

Apart from the crucial distinction between being 'inhabited' (*occupied*) rather than 'habituated' (*preoccupied*) by thoughts (Camilleri 2013d: 46–8), Varley refers to an aesthetic equivalent of an internal focus in a primary task

Attentional Focus in Performance 71

in sports: *thinking about the score*. The score, which in Odin Teatret refers to the design, details, dynamism, and organicity of an actor's sequence of actions in a performance (Barba [1993] 1995: 122; see also Chapter 3), implies the kind of behaviour that can be aligned with the automatization of practised sequences by elite athletes. In other words, like the guidance in sports training, Varley directs herself to 'not think about the score' with the aim of facilitating the flow of her performing.

As elaborated further in Chapter 6, compared to its desirable status in sports, a great deal of the bad press given to 'automaticity' in aesthetic performance is related to issues of terminology rather than to some unbridgeable discrepancy, particularly in the context of the professional practices discussed here. This is especially the case when considering that practices of mindfulness, which have currency in aesthetic performance (e.g. Zarrilli 2020: 11, 246), are increasingly featuring in sports training, including with reference to attentional focus and facilitating automaticity/flow (e.g. Moran 2012: 88; Brick et al. 2014: 120–1; Hutchinson 2018: 225–6).

Focused Distraction

Put simplistically, in raw terms that expose potential subterranean connections, what epistemic actions in aesthetic performance and secondary tasks in sports do, then, is a kind of '*distraction*' from one's own performance *at the same time as* one is focused *in* performance. Viewed from this angle, is not the constructed 'personal reality' of Stanislavski's actor a form of second-nature automatized behaviour? That is, once the actor mines her personal memories and, through various *scaffolded epistemic* activities, re-works them creatively *in the laboratory* into the character being interpreted, she 'becomes' the character on stage. In these circumstances, the distinction between self and score is suspended, thus enabling the 'actor/role' fusion or 'third being' that Benedetti mentions 'whereby one's own life experiences become the experience of the character' (Benedetti 2000: 95). Moreover, the 'distortion or a loss of time awareness' in flow experiences (Jackson 1996: 77) and the backgrounding of one's perception of effort (Camilleri 2023) are other facets of the 'distraction' that shifts the doer's attention from reflective to embodied modalities during optimal performance.

An additional aspect to consider deals with the manner by which the two phenomena straddle the physical and mental dimensions of behaviour. While epistemic operations, as defined by Hirsh and Maglio, are *physical* actions aimed at improving one's computational processing, for aesthetic performers this also involves the deployment of *mental* qualities such as memories, imagination, and the multi-sensory visualization discussed earlier. When the psychological realist actor opens a door on stage, she is not simply handling a prop but a 'real' door within 'real' circumstances as constructed via the epistemic scaffolding of evoking, developing, and applying her personal memories. For example, she might focus on the ergonomic feel of the handle to unlock the belief that there is a potential threat on the other side of the door that corresponds to a specific moment in her childhood.

In this way, the modal shift of attention prompted and sustained by epistemic actions is intended to trigger a behavioural and phenomenological shift from 'acting' to 'doing', thus paralleling the conceptualization of imagery as a 'quasi-perceptual phenomenological experience' evoked earlier in the context of sports. Viewed from this angle, therefore, epistemic actions serve to 'distract' actors – in part – from the fact that they are acting. Of course, this does not entail the loss of one's grasp on reality, i.e. an actor 'killing' someone on stage knows that she is 'acting killing'. In fact, as performance practitioner and performance studies scholar Richard Schechner clarifies, acting in such situations is better described as 'showing doing' (Schechner 2013: 28).

Regarding secondary tasks in athletic practice, their overtly distracting objective is evidently a *mental* strategy, even when accompanied by *physical* actions such as looking at a non-relevant point in the environment or saying a word when an action is executed (Cappuccio et al. 2019: 111). And yet the ultimate goal of such procedures is to enhance physical accuracy and effectiveness, almost as a side-effect, precisely by tasks designed to *distract* self-focused attention (Land 2007: 59). The question remains whether such strategies, especially of the non-sports-relevant variety usually employed in laboratory settings, are applicable in real-life competitive environments. Game or race situations, with their ever-changing ebb and flow of variables (including the pressure of high financial stakes and community expectations), demand considerable effort and ingenuity to generate secondary tasks, especially in the 'creative intuitive' sense of implicit know-how that facilitates 'the discovery of new combinations of elements' (Maldonato et al. 2019: 706; Moran 2012: 88). Consequently, rather than generic play creativity, specific instances could be targeted, for example, for set pieces like a penalty kick in the case of football. Speculatively, such real-life game situations could even be approached via an adapted version of Stanislavski's 'given circumstances' to enhance athletes' intuitive on-the-spur-of-the-moment and out-of-the-box dimensions of decision making (cf. Williams and Jackson 2019; Ford and O'Connor 2019).

Attentional Focus in Performance

Practice Insights

Other findings in Wulf's review of attentional focus and motor learning in sports that intersect with aesthetic processes include 'spread transmission' (my term), 'functional variability', and the 'distance effect'.

Spread transmission refers to the adverse muscular consequence of 'a performer's attentional focus on one part of the body [that] "spread[s]" to other muscle groups' (Wulf 2013: 84). This recalls a trait I often notice in novice participants during my physical theatre classes, e.g. how biting a lip, knitting eyebrows, tensing hands, or hunching shoulders whilst exercising or rehearsing can transfer ('spread') that tension to other parts of the body, including the voice. In some cases, I direct the trainee to 'untense' lips, shoulders, or the relevant part – which entails an internal focus when executing actions. Although the jury appears to be still out regarding the efficacy of dual task conditions for novices, the fact that 'inexperienced individuals demonstrate more effective performance when they focus on the skill (with either an external or internal focus), compared to when they are distracted by a secondary task, will be hardly surprising' (Wulf 2013: 92). At very early stages, motor learning is characterized by direct instructions to 'put your feet like this' and 'hold your hands like that'. However, aesthetic performance trainers may find it rewarding to explore different attentional options when transmitting fundamental skills such as body stances and alignment.

Other instances where I coach early learners to 'untense' a part of their body function along the lines of secondary tasks, e.g. if seeking to overcome a vocal obstacle, it is rarely useful to simply instruct 'clear your voice' or 'untense your voice' because the embodied knowledge to identify aspects of one's visceral body, let alone to intervene successfully, is still lacking. In such cases it may be more effective to direct the trainee to 'loosen shoulders' or 'imagine your voice is a feather' as a secondary task to the primary objective of singing a song or enunciating a text. Such strategies can tackle the issue without drawing attention to the obstacle itself, paradoxically 'distracting' the learner's focus from the source of the problem while addressing it practically.

Functional variability concerns movement kinematics or coordination on a higher level than the individual body part targeted by an exercise, i.e. when an external focus on one body part affects the organic totality of the body to achieve the desired result (Wulf 2013: 89). This characteristic resonates with the notion of 'sensorimotor exigencies' (discussed in Chapter 1) involving the automatic and non-conscious transferability of behavioural aspects from a particular context to another. After all, this is exactly the purpose

74   *Performer Training for Actors and Athletes*

of theatre training's adaptation of methods from martial arts, acrobatics, dance, and other somatic practices, i.e. not so much to enact the movement configurations of such skills (unless a performance score specifically demands it) but because their assimilation *informs*, at a deeper (embodied and non-conscious) level, a performer's scenic presence, hence improving the 'functional variability' of their behaviour.

Distance effect relates to the spatial extent between the agent and the object of her focus, i.e. whether distal or proximal. An accumulating number of studies shows that the advantage of external focus is enhanced when increasing the distance from the body, with some researchers arguing that 'a more distal focus makes the movement effect more easily distinguishable from the body movements that create the effect than a more proximal focus' (Wulf 2013: 97). One relevant example that Wulf mentions in this regard concerns long jump (Porter et al. 2012): focusing on leaping *towards* a target (distal) rather than *away from* the start lines (proximal) was found to be more effective.

Apart from reinforcing the value of having an external focus, the 'distance effect' suggests ways of experimenting with the practitioner's spatial awareness, including with reference to one's own sphere of movement influence, or the kinesphere as developed by dance artist and theorist Rudolf Laban (1879–1958). The kinesphere, which is actually more elliptic than spherical due to the body's constitution, defines 'the sphere around the body whose periphery can be reached by easily extended limbs without stepping away from that place which is the point of support when standing on one foot' (Laban [1939] 1966: 10). This space around the body moves as soon as the practitioner shifts her weight. It is also the first area of movement exploration before going into 'space in general'. In the short film on 'Awareness' of the *Physical Actor Training: An Online A–Z* (Allain et al. 2018), I demonstrate a related exercise loosely inspired by Laban's kinesphere. The purpose of this exercise, which is explained in more detail in the Conclusion, is to develop what can be called a 360-degree psychosomatic awareness, precisely by playing with distances *within* the 'sphere' by reaching out with different parts of the body. Apart from overall awareness and body conditioning for actors, athletes might also find such exercises useful as a form of cross-training, not only to target specific areas or dynamics but as a kind of physical meditation or mindfulness practice for flow capacity purposes.

These three aspects of attentional focus in sports can enhance the variety and, more importantly, the epistemic function of existing exercises for aesthetic performers. By combining dynamic perception (internal/external focus), use of imagination (e.g. inhabiting a sphere), and physical activity, such attentional strategies nurture a mental agility that is important to the awareness of actors and dancers as exemplified by Zarrilli's aesthetic inner bodymind. With regard to athletes, the insight provided by aesthetic processes can fine-tune interventions in the creative and intuitive dimensions associated with automatic unconscious reactions.

Cross-Sectional Perspectives for Actors and Athletes

Following this chapter's deliberations, the apparent resonance between internal/external attentional focus in sports and inner/outer action in aesthetic performance does not seem to stretch beyond a superficial terminological affinity. For in the case of aesthetic practice, epitomized by psychological realist processes but applicable to other genres, a performer can have an inner action (e.g. a specific memory) with an external focus (e.g. a door handle of the set). To be more precise, an actor can engage an external focus in a performance score that is *based on* and *sustained by* a composite or montage of inner actions. This means that the internal/external qualities of attentional focus and actions are not mutually exclusive of each other and can feature in various permutations with difference nuances. For example, an aesthetic outer action (such as a vocal or movement score) with an external focus prioritizes optimal technical execution, perhaps at the risk of not connecting (emotionally) with audiences if the artist's inner/imaginative process is lacking. Furthermore, the same outer action with an internal focus (that controls and regulates one's execution of action) is bound to create, as Varley notes, 'a separation within', i.e. between the individual and the performer ([1995] 2021: 215). The other combination available, an inner action (e.g. a memory) with an inner focus (on one's movement), marks an introspective and minimalist activity that can function as meditational training rather than as public performance in front of an audience.

From an athletic perspective, unless one is interested in increasing muscular mass (i.e. hypertrophy), the recommended approach is overwhelmingly in favour of external focus. Another possible exception concerns very early learners where an internal/skill focus characterizes the basic execution of actions, mainly to understand the mechanics involved. For instance, the first sessions of learning how to ride a bike are marked by an internal '*how-to*' attentional focus: how to sit, how to balance, how to pedal, how to change gears, and so on. With practice, one learns '*how to* let go'

76   *Performer Training for Actors and Athletes*

of micro-managing one's actions. When this happens, one no longer thinks about '*how to* ride a bike' but directs their attention externally: intentionally, distractedly, or both in the sense of Brick et al.'s (2014) 'active distraction' as discussed in Chapter 1.

But can athletes develop the equivalent of an aesthetic performer's 'inner action'? Although some aspects of inner action overlap with dimensions that are familiar to athletes, like the kind of strong motivation that emerges from life experiences, it is not the same thing as fostering a parallel *practice* of meditation, memories, and imagination to condition the individual's intentionality, agency, and therefore quality of actional execution in performance. Pragmatically speaking, it may be more appealing for athletes to concentrate on enhancing their competitive abilities, even though recovery or rest periods can be optimally deployed for such purposes. Any practice that endeavours to holistically improve the individual's wellbeing, whether physical or mental, quotidian or professional, has its benefits, and this includes 'inner action'.

Of course, there is no one-size-fits-all formula, not only because individuals are different but also because it depends on the nature of the sport, including whether it is intensively or minimally physical, or whether it is a solo or group discipline. An adapted 'inner action' approach to athletic practice can possibly draw on equivalents that already serve as supplementary practice in exceptional circumstances, such as assisting rehabilitation from injuries or maintaining a level of fitness (mental as well as physical) as acknowledged by an English Premiership footballer with regard to weekly online yoga sessions during the first Covid lockdown (Robertson 2020). In this regard, Roberto Baggio, the elite Italian footballer from the late 1980s and 1990s, epitomizes the value of inner strength – which he developed via Buddhist meditational practice – to cope with psychological frailty on and off the field (Baggio 1996).

A more sophisticated version of inner action for athletes that, like a Stanislavskian actor, builds on multi-sensory associations from memories and imagination to boost motivation and to support, drive, or enhance outer action, can provide the extremely fine cutting edge between two equally prepared individuals or teams, whether it serves to stimulate a person more optimally or bind a group even closer. In certain cases, especially those reliant on endurance, it can function as 'active distraction', including to reduce the perception of effort as discussed in Chapter 3.

Ultimately, however, the key difference between aesthetic and athletic performers remains the question of interpretation and expression of movement, which goes beyond the execution of action. At virtuosic levels that overlap with optimal experience, this difference is potentially

Attentional Focus in Performance 77

blurred when a kind of creative automaticity takes over and saturates the individual's performance both technically (as peak performance) and phenomenologically (as flow). The following chapter develops this and related aspects of the discussion with reference to other mind–body dimensions in athletic and aesthetic performance, specifically in the context of planning and strategy.

3

Maintaining the Pace:
Action Planning for Performance

This chapter develops the discussion about the *mind–body–world relationalities* of athletic and aesthetic processes, examining in more depth the paradoxical interplay between attention and automaticity in performance as identified so far in Part I. To this end, psychological and physiological aspects related to conscious and non-conscious processing are explored with regard to two major outlooks in sports science: the central governor theory and the psychobiological model of perceived effort. The argument is illustrated and elaborated with reference to pacing in endurance sports and to its proposed adaptation for aesthetic practices. In fusing action with strategic planning, pacing marks more structured psycho/physical dimensions that build on the movement cognitions and their mobilization in attentional focus as considered in Chapters 1 and 2 respectively.

Central Governor and Anticipatory Regulation

The name of the 'central governor' theory itself, as adapted and developed for endurance exercise by scientist and physician Tim Noakes, might be enough to straighten the backs of aesthetic performers who reject the notion of a dominant mind over a submissive body. But Noakes's hypothesis, which echoes a similar idea by 1922 Nobel laureate in Physiology or Medicine Archibald Vivian Hill (Hill et al. 1924: 163, 166), is not the sports science version of the Cartesian cogito that consciously controls the body.

Although the notion of a 'governing' entity implies a duality between the governor and the governed – specifically between the central nervous system (CNS) and peripheral organs – Noakes's theory could be viewed as a neurophysiological version of embodied cognition. It might even come across as 'too psychophysical' for practitioners who foreground and privilege the role of the physical body. For as a science expert in exercise physiology, and as an experienced ultra/marathon runner himself, Noakes operates from a materialistic/medical and practical/sports context that locates the

80 *Performer Training for Actors and Athletes*

central governor in the *brain* as an integral part of the body, rather than the Cartesian *mind* that rationalizes experience premeditatively and in isolation, almost irrespective of the vessel/vassal body.

Noakes's central governor involves a brain mechanism that regulates the intensity of physical exercise so that the body's homeostasis (i.e. its internal physical and chemical stability) is not threatened by prolonged strenuous activity (Noakes et al. 2001). The governor functions via the CNS by reducing the neural recruitment of muscle fibres, thus causing the sensation of fatigue, which in turn decreases the intensity of exertion with the purpose of maintaining homeostatic levels (Noakes et al. 2004; Noakes et al. 2005). What makes this theory potentially more body-centred than the most ardent psychophysical practitioners would wish is that the central governor does not operate entirely on a conscious, voluntary level. It can even override explicit conscious control, thus marking a form of physiological automaticity to safeguard its integrity. For example, deep into a high intensity or durational exercise, and even in moments when a runner or cyclist *wants* (and therefore, *intends*) to increase her pace, fewer muscles may be contracting, thus forcing the body to slow down to maintain temperature, heart rate, hydration, blood circulation, and other aspects below a critical point. As Alex Hutchinson observes:

> We have special nerve fibers that send information from the muscles to the brain about pressure, heat, damage, metabolic disturbances, and any number of other data points, and we integrate this information in our actions without even realizing it. Trying to make a clean divide between "brain fatigue" and "muscle fatigue," in other words, is inevitably an oversimplification, because they're inseparably linked.
>
> (Hutchinson 2018: 111)

Although such homeostatic disturbances are more likely in practices like running than in impact-free activities such as cycling or skiing (Hutchinson 2018: 111), let alone in traditional psychological realist acting (although intense and durational physical theatre and dance performances can be affected), their existence and potential activation sheds nuanced light on fundamental aspects of behavioural automaticity and body–mind relationality.

Noakes and his collaborators refer to this cautionary mechanism, which is triggered by the central governor well in advance to avoid 'catastrophic physiological failure', as 'anticipatory regulation'. Ross Tucker, a former student and then collaborator of Noakes, has suggested that Borg's index of subjective perception of effort during exercise, the RPE (rate of perceived

Action Planning for Performance

exertion), holds the key to the 'anticipatory regulation of performance' (Tucker 2009: 392). The RPE Scale was developed by psychophysicist Gunnar Borg (1927–2020) to measure the intensity of physical activity. The scale is used in many scientific studies and by various clinicians, especially when dealing with muscular, cardiac, and respiratory issues, but it features 'particularly in the field of sports medicine, where it is used by trainers to plan the intensity of training regimes, and in the workplace [...] to assess the exertion used in manual handling and physically active work' (Williams 2017: 404). In the context of endurance practices such as long-distance running, it articulates the effort that athletes feel when running.

The RPE constitutes a scale of 6–20, using verbal anchors from 'extremely light' on scale 7 to 'extremely hard' on scale 19 (Borg 1982: 378; Borg 1998: 30-1). This was subsequently developed by Borg himself to form a category ratio (CR) scale from 1 to 10, the Borg CR10, starting from '0 Nothing at all' and '0.5 Extremely weak (just noticeable)', all the way through '5 Strong (heavy)', '10 Extremely strong (almost max)', and the off-scale '* Maximal' (Borg 1982: 380; Borg 1998: 41). According to Borg, while the RPE enables the comparison of its values to 'such physiological measurements as heart rate (HR) and oxygen consumption ($\dot{V}O_2$)', the Borg CR10 scale is 'not determined by the form of any physiological functions or other measurements of exercise intensity, but by *internal psychophysical criteria*' (1998: 13, emphasis added). In other words, the original scale serves the more objective analyses involving testing, predictions, and prescriptions of perceived exertion, particularly (but not exclusively) by clinicians and coaches, whereas the CR10 is 'especially suitable for determining other subjective symptoms [of perceived effort], such as breathing difficulties, aches, and pain' (Borg 1982: 380; Camilleri 2023).

According to Tucker, in providing the 'biological link between the subjective [i.e. psychological] sensation of effort and the physiological [i.e. physical] changes occurring during exercise', the RPE potentially holds the key to regulating exercise performance and pacing strategy (2009: 392). Tucker posits the existence of a 'template RPE' – a theoretical construct that is generated from previous experience and from knowledge of the forthcoming exercise – against which the conscious/actual RPE is continuously compared during the activity (395). The past/future axes of accomplished/anticipated effort that this internal RPE represents is Tucker's explanation of how 'the brain knows in advance to slow you down before catastrophe strikes' (Hutchinson 2018: 210). And it does so automatically and unconsciously, from the very beginning of an endurance activity like a long run. As such, Tucker's model:

incorporates anticipatory/feedforward as well as feedback components, using an expectation of exercise duration *to set an initial work rate* and to generate what has been termed a subconscious "template" for the rate of increase in the RPE. During exercise, afferent feedback [transmission of sensory impulses from peripheral organs to the CNS] from numerous physiological systems is responsible for the generation of the conscious RPE, which is continuously matched with the subconscious template by means of *adjustments in power output*. This subjective rating is biologically linked, allowing pacing strategy to be adjusted to prevent catastrophic changes in the monitored physiological variables (homeostats).

(Tucker 2009: 400, emphasis added)

The implications of such a mechanism can be revealing for aesthetic performance. The idea of a performer's internalized template is discussed later in the chapter in the context of theatre scores and dance choreographies, i.e. of an embodied mental structure shaped by one's experience and expectations, that is continuously modulated during an activity and that serves as a dynamic reference against which to gauge and pace one's own performance. That such processes associated with the central governor are not always fully conscious or voluntary marks the main difference with another 'brain' perspective from sports science.

Psychobiological Model

Noakes's theory, like that of Hall's before him, is contested by the 'muscle' viewpoint that regulation by fatigue occurs as a result of homeostatic failure in locomotor muscles, i.e. due to a mechanical breakdown of the exercising (peripheral) muscles caused by inadequate oxygen (lactic acid build-up) or total energy depletion in the over-worked muscles. After all, the fact that 'catastrophic physiological failure' sometimes occurs in athletes indicates that the central governor can be overridden or that it does not always work. On this point, perspectives from embodied cognition, which reject the notion of a controller, do not ascribe muscle control to 'a program that the nervous system executes' but as emergent from 'tight interactions among the body, the nervous system, and the environment' (Shapiro and Spaulding 2019: 7). However, this does not necessarily conflict with Noakes's stance. Noakes's hypothesis has a lot going for it, including the emphasis on how the body functions (which necessarily

Action Planning for Performance

implicates the CNS), especially in extreme endurance conditions (which inevitably involves the environment).

My interest in outlooks such as Noakes's is to shed intersectional light on the bodyworld of athletic and aesthetic performers (i.e. their constitutive *body–mind–world* relational assemblages), with particular emphasis on what has tended to be overlooked in the endeavour to foreground the body: the role and contribution of the mind in performing bodies. As argued in the Introduction, the concept of bodyworld brings body and environment together on the psychophysical and embodied cognition assumption that body and mind are one and that the next binary to deconstruct is the human–non-human divide (see also Camilleri 2019: xi, xv, 177).

The psychobiological model of endurance performance by sports psychologist and scientist Samuele Marcora integrates exercise physiology, motivation psychology, and cognitive neuroscience (Marcora 2022). Although like Noakes he proposes a brain-centred outlook, with several overlapping features regarding the bigger picture of effort and fatigue, there are some significant operational differences. Before delving into these resonances and contrasts with the aim of shedding further light on *embodied brain processes* and their relation to performers' bodyworld, it is important to clarify potential fundamental misunderstandings that risk arising due to different terminological and conceptual assumptions by athletic and aesthetic practitioners and scholars.

The nomenclature of a 'brain-centred' perspective in sports science does not carry the same connotations that it does in theatre and dance studies. Since at least their explicit emergence in the second half of the twentieth century (but also before that as we saw with Antonin Artaud in the Introduction), studies in aesthetic practices like theatre, dance, and performance have gone through a 'psychophysical consequence' in the so-called 'turn to practice' (Schatzki et al. 2001). That is, the *foregrounding of practice* inevitably emphasized *body processes*, both of which entailed the rejection of Cartesian dualism that privileged the rational mind over the brute body (Schatzki 2001: 16). The emergence of 'theatre studies' as a distinct academic discipline with dedicated university departments that focused on the *staging* of theatre productions (including their histories and processes of training, composition, technology, and reception), rather than on the *literary* qualities of play texts, is but one feature of this turn to practice (Nelson 2013: 12–16). Prior to this late twentieth-century development, 'drama' existed along with poetry and prose writing as literary appreciation in language departments. As I argued elsewhere: 'Psychophysicality, in discourse if not in practice, is an important battle that has been won. The concepts of "psychophysicality" and "bodymind" now occupy the same space that the unconscious, the sign system, and social class structure enjoy in other spheres of human knowledge: we no longer need to justify their discursive existence' (Camilleri 2013d: 30). In this context, therefore, the notion of a 'brain-centred' perspective is a regressive step, redolent of Cartesian overtones of mind supremacy.

Conversely, in the body-saturated context of sports, especially in athletics and more so in endurance activity, a 'brain-centred' outlook marks an appreciation of the mental and psychological *along with* the physical and physiological. Such an understanding considers athletic practice not only as a question of muscles and biology but, instead, it also incorporates mental capacities in meaningful ways. As sports writer and coach Matt Fitzgerald argues, 'many aspects of endurance performance that were always presumed to be biological in nature are now known to be mind-based'. For example, it is the *psychology* of 'feeling thirsty' that slows down athletes rather than the *biology* of dehydration (Fitzgerald 2016: 8). This is where Marcora comes in with his 'psychobiological' approach.

Although Marcora's 'psychobiological' has evident overtones with 'psychophysical', his understanding is closer to Gunnar Borg's than Phillip Zarrilli's deployment of the term. Borg uses 'psychophysical' in the scientific 'psychophysics' sense that studies the perceptual relationality between stimulus and sensation (e.g. Borg 1982; Borg 1998: 13), which is distinct from its phenomenological application in theatre and performance as the integration of outer/physical and inner/psychic action in which body–mind dualism is overcome (Zarrilli 2020: 9–12). Still, both cases underline an *organic* connectivity that indexes mind and body *integrity* rather than merely a bridged separability. For what binds mind and body together is the brain, a *physical organ* that, along with the spinal cord, makes up the central nervous system that coordinates and influences the activity of all parts of the body.

Fitzgerald argues that emphasizing the brain in sports brings body and mind together rather than the contrary (2016: 12). From this viewpoint, a sports practice that, in addition to the requisite body techniques, cultivates *physically* what Fitzgerald calls 'mental fitness' is better equipped to accomplish a task more optimally. Such an outlook reads like the sports equivalent of Zarrilli's conceptualization of the 'aesthetic inner bodymind' that performers nurture in training and which shapes the 'aesthetic outer body' offered to the spectators' gaze (Zarrilli 2009: 58; see also Chapter 1). This comparison is even more apt when recalling the appreciation that practices like mindfulness are increasingly enjoying in athletic preparation (see Chapter 2; Hutchinson 2018: 225–6).

Action Planning for Performance   85

Perception of Effort

At the heart of Marcora's psychobiological model is *perception of effort*, not actual effort per se but one's *feeling* or *sense* of it. The difference between actual/biological and perceived/psychological effort has crucial implications: it implies that an individual's performance exceeds the mere sum of her physical capacities considered separately. Anything that conditions the feeling of effort is bound to affect one's endurance: from *continuous training* itself, that decreases the sense of effort (Fitzgerald 2016: 10), to positive *self-talk* as encouraging stimulant (Hutchinson 2018: 260), to strategically *enacting smiles or frowning* to untense or maximize muscle contraction (Brick et al. 2018: 26; see also Chapter 5), to *swishing and spitting* energy drink rather than swallowing it (Brietzke et al. 2019: 65), thus impacting the feeling of thirst rather than hydration (for it is 'thirst, not dehydration, [that] increases your sense of perceived effort and in turn causes you to slow down', Hutchinson 2018: 174), to the comfort qualities of *shoe design* (Liu et al. 2021: 233), to the at once distractive and stimulating effect of listening to *music* (Patania et al. 2020: 5), to post-workout *ice-baths* that athletes overwhelmingly swear by even if scientific evidence is ambiguous about their benefit (Leeder et al. 2012: 233), to *placebos, self-belief* (Hutchinson 2018: 250–3), and other elements.

Although both Noakes and Marcora emphasize the role played by the perception of effort in athletic performance, hence the methodological deployment of the Borg RPE in their respective studies, the main bone of contention concerns the *endpoint of activity* when pushed to the extreme such as in endurance situations. Contrary to Noakes, whose central governor stands for an unconscious mechanism that regulates homeostasis via sensory feedback from the 'subconscious brain', Marcora argues for 'voluntary control' by the 'conscious brain' or perceived exertion (Marcora 2008: 930; Marcora 2009). Although the two scientists have argued about this aspect, Noakes admits that only 'minor differences' separate them because both agree on the decisive part played by the brain rather than on the historical emphasis on locomotor organs to limit exercise performance (Noakes and Tucker 2008: 933; Hutchinson 2018: 70).

Discussing Marcora's model in the context of related studies by exercise physiologists, Fitzgerald illustrates at once the proximity and distance with Noakes's position:

> Except in the case of reflex actions, all muscle work begins with an act of conscious willing. This command originates in the brain's motor cortex and supplementary motor area. Scientists are able to measure the intensity of these commands, and this measurement is referred to

as movement-related cortical potential (MRCP). Marcora has shown that MRCP and perception of effort are high when subjects exercise at maximum intensity and also that they increase covariantly when exercise of lower intensity is performed for a long period of time. This is compelling evidence that *perceived effort is indeed related to brain activity, not muscle activity.*

(Fitzgerald 2016: 47, emphasis added)

The key point that links *perceived effort* with *brain activity* is shared by Marcora and Noakes – what separates them are their respective *explanations for this relationship*: Marcora argues that 'we pace ourselves to keep the effort manageable, and quit when it gets higher than we're willing to tolerate. In contrast, Noakes [...] sees the sense of effort as a conscious manifestation of hardwired neural circuitry that kicks in to hold us back from the precipice' (Hutchinson 2018: 210). It appears to be a case of different constellation patterns from the same group of stars. But what if it is possible to hypothesize a composite picture or an overlay of the two constellations?

Following his separate interviews with the two of them, Hutchinson appears to make a case for a nuanced appreciation that brings both models closer together:

Marcora does indeed argue that the decision to speed up, slow down, or stop is always conscious and voluntary. But such "decisions," he acknowledges, can be effectively forced on you by an intolerably high sense of effort. [...] Noakes and his colleagues, on the other side, don't dispute the importance of effort, motivation, and conscious decision making. When you run a marathon, it's not the central governor that prevents you from sprinting for the first 100 meters [...].

(Hutchinson 2018: 70)

Although Noakes and Marcora go into some length to distinguish their approaches (Marcora 2008; Noakes and Tucker 2008), the details become almost irrelevant when considered in the light of their principal convergence, *that perceived effort is related to brain not muscle activity.* Indeed, despite the divergences that imply different ways of training – especially with Marcora's ongoing development of brain endurance programmes that target mental resilience via durational and repetitive cognitive tasks and puzzles (Hutchinson 2018: 212–27) – the *action implications* of their convergence are more intriguing. In other words, what does the brain-regulated perception of effort, *which conditions actual effort,* say about the resultant performance and the athlete's control over it? The complex connection between focused attention and automaticity is brought to the fore once again.

Action Planning for Performance

Tucker's formulation of anticipatory regulation overlaps with elements of Brick, MacIntyre, and Campbell's (2014) updated model of associative attentional focus discussed in Chapter 1. The connection involves the anticipatory regulation's mainly *non-conscious processing* of 'internal sensory monitoring' (which deals with effort *sensations* such as breathing, muscle soreness, thirst, and perspiration) and 'active self-regulation' (which concerns technique and strategy, including pacing) (Brick et al. 2014: 111, 113). Conversely, Brick et al.'s (2014) revised categories of 'active distraction' and 'involuntary distraction' impacts not so much one's actual effort but its *perception*, in the process mitigating the feeling of exertion, enabling the individual to push harder for longer, thus enhancing performance.

The picture painted in this cross-lighting of perspectives is intriguingly paradoxical: on the one hand, *a sensorial monitoring that operates unconsciously* via the nervous system, and, on the other hand, *a 'distractive' focus* that takes one's mind off the processing of effort. If anything, this image of extreme performance, which reflects the fuller range available to the performer as much as it situates that same potential in every action, is one of *constantly shifting modes of attention that bleed into each other*: consciousness and automaticity, focus and distraction. This modulating condition is something that aesthetic practitioners can relate to, especially those who advocate a fine balance between highly technical training and a kind of letting go in performance – almost similar to the trance-like flow of optimal experience – as marked by Grotowski's 'passive readiness', Lindh's 'disinterested act', and Zarrilli's 'chiasmatic body', all evoked in Chapter 1.

An intersectional perspective of this kind, that cuts across different strands of research, underlines the elusiveness of a grand unified theory. More importantly, it foregrounds the performer's focus as a site of multi-tiered and multi-directional body–mind interactions. A simplistic understanding of an individual's intentions, imagination, or even desire and motivation is not enough. Indeed, the sense of human agency that comes with intentionality, imagination, and aspiration does not account for the often non-conscious but equally decisive dimensions of physiological processes and mutually shaping relations with the environment.

Pacing

What does the composite picture about attentional focus and effort perception in sports say to aesthetic performers? Actors and dancers are often asked to be at one with their actions and to be free from extraneous thoughts that distract them from the task at hand. But *how* and *on what* does one focus during the work? What does one materially *do* when

88   *Performer Training for Actors and Athletes*

focusing? A subtler appreciation of the variables and complexities at play, such as the ones explored so far in this book, while not necessarily directly applicable, can serve to defamiliarize ingrained assumptions and widen the range of training options for aesthetic performers. Accordingly, the rest of the chapter deals with a concrete example of what sports knowledge can contribute to aesthetic performance. In the light of the above brain-oriented discussion on attention, focus, effort, and perception, *pacing* in athletic practice is contemplated in view of its proposed equivalent in aesthetic processes. Within this frame, pacing is considered as a sophisticated instance of *planning by* and *of action.*

Pacing marks an intrinsically and explicitly psychophysical (or psychobiological) dimension that brings strategy and action together in the ongoing activity of monitoring and adjustment. In performance, one is only ever out of pacing when one stops at the end of a task, and even then it usually marks but a phase in a longer itinerary that involves other events. Although pacing is not technically necessary or equally important for all sports, all human practices (including daily life) require what may otherwise be called the organization and management of resources, making sure that one has the capacity and energy for the task ahead, especially if it entails depth and/or duration of engagement. Pacing is essential for running because, as Hutchinson observes, 'any task lasting longer than a dozen or so seconds requires decisions, whether conscious or unconscious, on how hard to push and when' (2018: 11), precisely because it demands strategic use of one's resources with respect to environmental factors (e.g. whether uphill or downhill, road or trail, sunny or raining), other competitors, and ultimately oneself.

Fitzgerald is even more specific about the time of physiological resistance when he argues that any race longer than 30 seconds requires the individual to hold back:

> Athletes are conscious of their effort in shorter races, of course, but because they know their suffering will end quickly they do not *use this perception to control their pace*, which is constrained only by their physical capacity. But when an athlete starts a race that he knows will last longer than 30 seconds, he holds back just enough that his perceived effort limit is not reached until he is at the finish line. That is the art of pacing.
>
> (Fitzgerald 2016: 67, emphasis added)

Although the intensity mentioned here marks an extreme form of engagement, including the slower but durational ones associated with

Action Planning for Performance 89

endurance practices, as observed on various occasions in this book, such extremity puts in higher relief existing conditions and mechanisms that are operative in human behaviour more generally.

When an activity is low intensity, like climbing a couple of stairs or walking around in a shopping mall, the fact that this mechanism is not perceptually foregrounded does not mean that it is not active – it operates in the background of consciousness and comes to the fore if there is a change in circumstances, like arriving at a long flight of stairs and one assesses (rapidly and often unconsciously) the effort/capacity required to climb them or use the lift or escalator instead. Of course, this cycle or four-way pattern of monitoring–assessment–decision–action, which can be aligned with a sense of pacing, is more refined in athletes because it has been experienced and worked upon at length, and can thus be used as a measure to calibrate (*control*) one's reserves and expenditure of energy. This is especially the case with endurance practices because, in addition to discipline-specific techniques, they thematize the organization and management of resources (mental, physical, emotional), which is what pacing is about.

Aesthetic performances, like typical theatre pieces that last between 30 to 90 minutes (but also for shorter productions, and even more so for longer presentations like classical plays, musicals, opera, and the occasional multiple-hours project), come with a comparable 'energy management' that can be aligned with pacing. Although not all aesthetic productions need the performer to remain on stage for the entire duration of the piece, and making allowance for the different stylistic genres and roles (e.g. ranging from physically engaging ensemble theatre to multiple minor parts in a realist play), the notion of *pacing in aesthetic performance* is highly relevant because it directly concerns the *performer's 'presence'*.

Scenic presence is the medium of expression in aesthetic performance, it is the language of the message and, in postdramatic productions that draw attention to their methods of construction, can be the language–message itself (Lehmann 2006: 18–21). Therefore, even if an actor has a brief role in a theatre/dance piece, she is required – very relevantly in this context – to *hit the ground running*, because her input is part of a bigger picture. It is like listening to an orchestra and one of the instruments, however minor, is slightly out of tune: its *presence/performance* draws attention to itself. One way of hitting the ground running in aesthetic performance, which requires experience and know-how *of managing one's resources*, is to be already 'in character' before first entering the scene and/or when one is temporarily off stage during a performance. As such, pacing is an ongoing plan(ning) of action that occurs *in* performance.

Aesthetic Pacing

The conceptualization of 'aesthetic pacing' highlights the potential benefits of deploying insights from athletics and sports science to aesthetic performance and vice versa. Aesthetic performance, like its athletic counterpart, is constituted of specialized behaviour structured around certain rules within set parameters. Consequently, both partake of dimensions that they share in common, including movement patterns and rhythms, duration of activity, intensity and modulation of energy, and segmentation (e.g. episodes or scenes in aesthetic performance, and periods, halves, sets, or rounds in sports). It is in the inflected similarities and differences between the two camps – which individually are far from homogeneous – that the potential for insight resides. In this regard, pacing is ideally placed because, in marking the quality of habitation of an athletic or aesthetic event (i.e. its execution or interpretation), it brings together the different elements of a performance structure. I return to 'aesthetic pacing' in the Conclusion to highlight an important aspect of the habitational modality associated with *via athletae* in the Introduction. Here I elaborate on some of the practicalities and implications of the concept.

One difference between athletic and aesthetic performances involves the extent of structured organization. In the great majority of cases, theatre and dance productions follow more or less *fixed* configurations and sequences of actions that are structured on scaffolded cues of varying complexity. The fixity of these arrangements in turn allows multiple interactions to occur between several performers as well as facilitates scenic effects like lights, projections, and sound. Such concatenated organization enables the performance to be repeated with a high level of consistency every night, sometimes more than once daily and with different performers.

Much of this structured and relational framework also applies for the more experimental performances that allow varying degrees of improvisation. In these cases, the relatively unstructured elements (e.g. impromptu interactions with fellow performers or the audience; see also Case Study 4 in Chapter 6) are framed and contained within the overall arrangement. This includes seemingly 'open' improvisations that are guided (i.e. 'structured') by elements such as themes, objects, instruments, location, or even the technical background and/or number of performers (e.g. a duo triggers different dynamics than a trio). 'Free' improvisations of this kind (which generally feature in the training, composition, and rehearsal processes of some productions) are, by nature, occasional and special events because if repeated regularly and at length they tend to adopt the unavoidably recurring elements as organizational structure.

Action Planning for Performance   91

The fixed structures in aesthetic performance, which allow a degree of freedom during their interpretation, are unlike group and solo sports such as football, basketball, tennis, and golf that, despite following prescribed rules and involving elements of repeated behaviour and automaticity, unfold in the style of an improvisation. Indeed, except for certain prescribed limits like duration (e.g. 90 minutes for a football match), no one game or match is like any other despite having the same players, location, and rules. At the other end on the sports spectrum, athletic practices like javelin/discus-throwing and long/high jumps entail precise 'choreographies' of action, i.e. they include a high level of fixed actions. What varies in these latter practices occurs on the level of individual styles and their extent to improve results. That these are almost invariably solo sports, and therefore restricting the complexity and quantity of variables in play, contributes to the choreographization of the athletic performance. Group sports that consist of very precise behavioural patterns, like rowing, involve repetition to such an extent that 'group work' amounts to *coordination of the same actions* by all.

Somewhere halfway on this spectrum of athletic possibilities lies running. Despite the relative freedom of the activity (in part ascribed to its simplicity in that anyone who walks can technically run), it involves a substantial degree of strategy: when to hold back, let go, push forward, maintain, overtake, or be overtaken, etc. In this scenario, pacing is queen, making it ideal for the purposes of application and adaptation because the variables in running are relatively minimal compared to other sports that demand more complex actions than putting one foot in front of another as fast and/or for as long as possible.

Similar to its athletic equivalent, aesthetic pacing entails overseeing and regulating processes, including internal/external monitoring and anticipatory/retrospective analysis. For a clearer picture of the aesthetic structures involved and to situate such processes and their component elements more concretely, Eugenio Barba's description of *score* in his theatre practice can be adopted as a model that applies more generally:

At Odin Teatret, the term *score* referred to:

[1]   the general design of the form in a sequence of actions, and the evolution of each single action (beginning, climax, conclusion);

[2]   the precision of the fixed details of each action as well as of the transitions connecting them (*sats* [impulse, readiness to react (Barba [1993] 1995: 54–9)], changes of direction, different qualities of energy, variations of speed);

[3]   the dynamism and the rhythm: the speed and intensity which regulated the *tempo* (in the musical sense) of a series of actions. This was the metre of the actions with their micro-pauses and decisions,

92   *Performer Training for Actors and Athletes*

the alternation of long or short ones, accented or unaccented segments, characterised by vigorous or soft energy;

[4]   the orchestration of the relationships between the different parts of the body (hands, arms, legs, feet, eyes, voice, facial expression).

(Barba 2010: 27–8; see also Barba [1993] 1995: 122, emphasis in the original)

Although all four aspects deal with the *manifestation* of a performance score, and therefore with its external dimension, it is possible to discern some subtle differences. The 'design', 'form', structure (beginning–middle–end) and 'fixed details' (including 'direction', 'quality', and 'variation' of energy) of Barba's first two points refer to the external characteristics or *shape* of an aesthetic performance score. Conversely, the 'dynamism', 'rhythm', and organicity ('orchestration') of the performer's actions in the remaining two points, although also manifested in behaviour, provide a window on the internal features that drive that external. If points (1) and (2) refer to the *idealized* structure of the score (what it *should look* like), points (3) and (4) mark its here-and-now *actualization* or *experience* (what it *feels* like). That is, 'what it feels like' for *the practitioner* when performing the score, but also – and crucially in the communicative context of aesthetic performance – what consequently conditions its reception by the *audience*. (More about sensory and emotional feeling in Part II.)

The feeling of motion and its organization in Barba's third point provides the key to the aesthetic pacing that – I am proposing – drives the score as a coherent and organic whole, translating it from the 'singular sameness' of the idealized structure to the 'different multiplicity' of the performed actualizations that audiences experience. It is precisely this *felt dynamism* that breathes life into the 'general design' and the 'fixed details [and] transitions' of the sequence of actions that constitute a performance score. It is also what enlivens and 'orchestrates the different parts of the body'. It is no coincidence that Barba associates this dynamism with 'the speed and intensity' that 'regulates' the tempo of the actions that *compose* the score as it is being performed. The overseeing and adjustment activities – whether conscious or otherwise – that accompany such 'regulation' resonates with a similar aspect in sports that relates to pacing: 'anticipatory regulation'.

Dynamic Modulation

Like a constellation in the sky, Fitzgerald draws the lines of connection between pacing, feeling, Marcora's perception of effort, and Noakes's and Tucker's anticipatory regulation, summarizing the salient points thus:

Action Planning for Performance

In endurance races, athletes pace themselves largely by feel. External feedback [...] may influence pacing, but it's an internal sense of the appropriateness of one's pace from moment to moment that has the first and final say in determining whether an athlete chooses to speed up, hold steady, slow down, or collapse into a lifeless heap. The scientific name for this pacing mechanism is *anticipatory regulation*. Its output is a continuously refreshed, intuition-like feeling for how to adjust one's effort in order to get to the finish line as quickly as possible. Its inputs are perception of effort, motivation, knowledge of the distance left to be covered, and past experience.

(Fitzgerald 2016: 46–7, emphasis in the original)

In view of the identification of anticipatory regulation as a pacing mechanism in athletics, I propose 'dynamic modulation' as a possible equivalent for aesthetic pacing.

The notion of 'dynamic modulation' builds on the concept of 'anticipatory regulation' from sports and that of 'modulation' from Zarrilli's model of performer experience and embodiment (see Chapter 1). Since 'regulation' may come across as too regimental in aesthetic performance contexts, with connotations of mechanistic and predetermined control, the preferred term 'modulation' is representative of those 'subtler/"inner" dimensions' that are cultivated in training for the benefit of performance (Zarrilli 2020: 31, 128). Indeed, Zarrilli's reading explicates 'a constantly shifting *tactical improvisation* modulating betwixt and between one's bodymind and its modes of engaging its own deployment in the score (physical and textual) during training and performance' (Zarrilli 2009: 60, emphasis in the original). To transpose Fitzgerald's words about pacing to an aesthetic context, Zarrilli's *constantly shifting modulation* is certainly informed by the individual's 'perception of effort, motivation, knowledge of the [score/choreography] left to be covered, and past experience'. As such, 'dynamic modulation' refers to an actor's or dancer's aesthetic and technical sensibility – a refined *awareness* – that monitors and adjusts internal/external action *across the duration of a performance*. Consequently, the phrases 'anticipatory regulation' and 'dynamic modulation' distinguish, as much as they mark the resonance, between processes of control (conscious or otherwise) in athletic and aesthetic practices respectively.

But do actors and dancers pace themselves when performing? As Barba's account of score exemplifies, the various layers involved and their inter-relationalities necessarily point to an organizing structure that serves as a plan of/for action. The mechanism or dynamics I am aligning with pacing, something that is hardly ever discussed directly in aesthetic performance

94 *Performer Training for Actors and Athletes*

and performer process, reflects the capacity of enacting or 'living through' this organizing arrangement of elements and dimensions. In marking the space of *how to?*, i.e. '*how to* deploy technique or manage race strategies or aesthetic scores?', pacing can be viewed as a second-order procedure or meta-approach that depends on – because it works with – other processes and aspects.

Theatre, dance, and other performers necessarily pace themselves on a somatic level, especially if a score is physically demanding in its entirety or in parts, including if it has any challenging vocal actions (text or song) that require reserves of breath and a suitable stance/support for their execution, thus needing advance preparation. What about emotional pacing? Do aesthetic performers pace themselves to peak at the right time and, equally important, in an appropriate way? It is worth exploring this question in the context of psychological realist acting where the representation of emotions – from the subtle to the potentially strident – is integral to the aesthetic event.

An actor's *building up to* a demanding emotional scene, that would otherwise be rendered mechanically flat or unconvincingly amplified, is a clear example of moment-to-moment planned and controlled pacing, however 'intuitive' it may be for some performers. Indeed, it is such pacing that facilitates the actor to 'let go' (to *flow*) at the right time. But emotional pacing can be located on subtler and more fundamental levels in realist drama, i.e. on the level of *how does an actor manage her own emotions* and *those of the role being portrayed?* This is an iteration of a question with a long history that, without going further back, can be dated to the nineteenth century. In this modern period, it starts with French philosopher Denis Diderot (1713–1784), who, in the posthumously published essay *Le Paradoxe sur le comédien* ('Paradox of the Actor', 1830), argued that great actors *do not experience the emotions* they display on stage. The debate continued with Stanislavski's lifetime research, spilling over into the twentieth century and is still highly influential today. Contrary to Diderot, Stanislavski emphasized the actor's *deep immersion* in the role, a becoming-one with it (Hodge 2010a: xix–xx; see also Chapter 2). The organizational question of *how to* calibrate such interplays between personal and portrayed emotions marks the modulation I am ascribing to aesthetic pacing. It is what enables an actor to enact emotions on stage.

From a Stanislavskian perspective, this modulating capacity permits an actor to actualize a character's 'through line', that is, not as a fragmented set of aims, emotions, and actions in any given unit, which is an important part of the rehearsal process, but to understand and embody the line that links all aspects together, if necessary reaching out to a time *before* the events in

Action Planning for Performance 95

a play (Aquilina 2016: 118), thus pushing (pacing) the character forward through the narrative:

> That inner line of effort that guides the actors from the beginning to the end of the play we call the *continuity* or the *through-going action*. This through line galvanizes all the small units and objectives of the play and directs them toward the super-objective. From then on they all serve the common purpose.
>
> (Stanislavski [1936] 1989: 296, emphasis in the original)

Stanislavski's choice of words is revealing: 'effort', 'from beginning to the end', 'continuity', 'galvanizes', and 'directs' all resonate strongly with a conceptualization of aesthetic pacing. It is in this sense that an actor's through line, which incorporates what amounts to *a character's emotional itinerary*, corresponds to strategy or game plan in athletic events.

Calibrating Inner Action

The calibration or aesthetic pacing of enacted emotions in performance is integral to what in Chapter 2 is discussed as the 'inner action' of memories, imagination, and other phenomena that subtend the 'outer action' seen on stage by audiences. From the present chapter's perspective, an actor's inner action consists of both an expansive understanding of Stanislavski's 'inner line [or sense] of effort' (i.e. the through line that brings elements together), and Fitzgerald's 'internal sense of the appropriateness of one's pace' (as reflected in an athlete's RPE). This internal emotional/perceptual dimension, which contributes to mental state, necessarily involves a performer's physical capacity to execute the score.

However, before it is *actualized* in performance, the score exists as an *idealized* structure, a kind of memorized template in the performer's awareness, like Tucker's non-conscious 'template RPE' that regulates exercise intensity and pacing strategy. This template, against which the conscious/actual RPE is continuously compared *during* the activity, includes not only the performer's assimilation of the complex components featured in Barba's description of a score, but also all the coordination cues with fellow performers and the technical team managing the production. As such, the internal dimension involves a (memorized and embodied) plan of action of 'what's coming next?' that enables the score to be performed bit by bit, segment by segment, with the transitions in between. This materialized translation of *a plan of action* into *actualized action* is driven/galvanized by a performer's aesthetic pacing.

In his examination of 'strategy' and 'monitoring skills' by runners, metacognition researcher John Nietfeld includes the category of *planning* as 'thoughts related to pre-race preparations' that condition an individual's psychological and action processes (2003: 313). This type of pre-event planning informs the template RPE with knowledge of the route and its duration. Moreover, it overlaps with and feeds into another category identified by Nietfeld: 'strategies that the runner employs during the competition' (313), which serve to fine-tune the plan (or template) as it is being actualized. Although not as tightly fixed as an aesthetic performance score, such metacognitive phenomena shed further light on the processes denoted by aesthetic pacing. In the current context, metacognition refers to the 'mental tactics that athletes employ to improve performance' (Nietfeld 2003: 307), especially those relating to race or run design, whether planned prior to or during an event.

Although pacing is manifested somatically, the emotional, strategic, imaginative, memories, and memorized aspects involved make of it an equally *metacognitive* phenomenon, and as such is optimally placed in discussions on psycho/physicality and body/mind. The mental dimension of aesthetic pacing that entails the planning of action concerns the actor's state/s of mind at various points in a performance, not as a singular or static state but as fluctuating and evolving towards a finishing line. Indeed, pacing starts with a mental preparation and readiness that overlaps with what Fitzgerald calls 'bracing oneself' ahead of a demanding task (2016: 49–50), and that becomes more pronounced with longer distances for endurance athletes.

To evoke my personal experience, whenever I run more than 30 km, I spend most of the week thinking and repeating to myself: '30, 30, 30' or whatever the number of kilometres I am aiming to run. This 'thinking' is not always intentional; it is frequently a background awareness that occasionally surfaces in the foreground as some kind of mantra. I now recognize this as preparation, as part of a planning process that operates along the lines of anticipatory regulation, which also serves to condition my perception of effort *ahead* of the event. For shorter distances (say, anything up to 15 km), the mechanism is more immediate in that I foreground the number during the day of or right before the run. A comparable feeling characterizes my experience of performing on stage, a mental preparedness that occurs in the final week or so. However, in this case, instead of numbers I have flashes in my consciousness of instances in the idealized/template score that require particular attention or which I enjoy and look forward to performing. Although these flashes may be 'unplanned', they are certainly reflective of the ongoing preparation or planning process of the performance.

Action Planning for Performance 97

Despite the fact that acting and dancing are not generally a solo endeavour, it is hardly contentious to claim that they are 'experienced' as such in terms of the intensity of presence on stage. That is, one has to be 'switched on' (engaged) even when supposedly doing 'nothing' because it contributes to the aesthetic occurrence/expression on stage. This phenomenological intensity parallels that of the solo practice of running, including when running in a group. Although the company of others might condition the perception of effort, making it more bearable, its accumulation eventually catches up with the individual. To this extent, athletes experience running always in centre stage – they are literally always *on the go*, never not doing anything. In contrast, team sports like football or rugby can involve moments or phases of relative passivity (e.g. when the ball is on the other side of the pitch) or deactivation (e.g. when there is a break in play due to an injury). That is, even when the players are focused on what is happening around them, their physical presence is not as activated as when the principal game device (the ball in this case) is in close proximity.

A general principle can be extracted from this football example to shed further light on attentional focus: the degree of voluntary activation and extent of psychophysical excitability is proportional to the proximity of the ball in team sports like football, rugby, water polo, baseball, and basketball. The closer to the ball, the more the individual is 'switched on'. This complements aspects of attentional focus that have already been discussed, especially Wulf's research on internal/body and external/environment focus and its proximal/distal variations (Chapter 2). With actors and dancers, however, as well as athletes like runners whose sport does not include an object, the individual is always *in proximity* to the main action, i.e. to *herself* as subject/object of performance. That this applies even when occupying a peripheral place in a group scene on stage or during a race goes some way in accounting for the intensity of felt experience, hence the imperative of pacing one's excitability and energy.

Grafting Insights

Although the implications of aesthetic pacing and dynamic modulation may not immediately result in much that is new for actors and dancers, they foreground a dimension that is often overlooked or assumed. Aesthetic performers are taught and learn techniques but are then expected to know *how to* breathe life into their performance, i.e. how to 'galvanize' and *pace* the elements at their disposal when enacting the *plan of action* that constitutes a score or choreography. However, becoming sensitized to pacing in theatre

98   *Performer Training for Actors and Athletes*

and dance contributes to the holistic and corporeal assimilation of these component parts also in psychological and emotional ways.

Performers, like other learners, assimilate elements in bits and pieces, gradually over time, which is similar to learning a language by progressing through the alphabet, words, phrases, and sentences before one starts talking or writing fluently (indeed, 'flowingly'). It is only with regular practice, during rehearsals and extended runs of a performance, that pacing is refined to an extent that any issues, however minimal, are flagged up and/or rectified during the activity. As a practice, then, pacing marks a second-order process that operates on and re-organizes existing material. From this angle, the planning of action entailed by aesthetic pacing is as much *technique* as it is *strategy*, once again straddling the physical/mental dimensions of embodied practices.

Can this second-order technique/strategy be trained? Or is it a matter that simply 'occurs' with practice and experience? It can be trained in so far as Zarrilli's subtle 'aesthetic inner bodymind', which is not a specific skill per se but a mode of awareness, can be trained, that is, via 'long-term, in-depth engagement in certain psychophysical practices or training regimes [such as] yoga, the martial arts, *butoh*, acting/performing per se [...] which engage the physical body and attention (mind) in cultivating and attuning both to subtle levels of experience and awareness' (Zarrilli 2009: 55). Considered in this light, aesthetic pacing can be nurtured quasi-indirectly because as a second-level process it relies on the extent and depth of first-level skills. What sports can contribute here, apart from other first-level practices like those listed by Zarrilli, are ways of organizing the pacing of aesthetic performance via the knowledge of capacities and mechanisms like attentional focus variations, anticipatory regulation (or dynamic modulation), and perception of effort.

To deploy Zarrilli's terms from phenomenology, thus grafting insights from sports science onto theatre and dance processes, aesthetic pacing can be viewed as the engagement *and* management of the 'aesthetic inner bodymind' *during* the presentation of the 'aesthetic outer body'. One way that this management occurs is through the *aesthetic modulation* or the ongoing monitoring–adjustment (which is not necessarily always conscious) of the performance in its *holistic integrity* rather than as a collection of units. In this scenario, the performer's bodyworld ability to *sense* conditions and alterations in oneself and the surrounding world is of paramount importance. Accordingly, following Part I's emphasis on the mental dimensions in the embodied performance of athletic and aesthetic practitioners, it is now time to turn our attention to the question of *feeling* and its attendant sensorial and emotional dimensions that condition perception and action.

Part II

Heart Matters

4

Feeling Performance:
Affect, Sensation, Emotion

Perception of effort emerges as a seminal aspect in Part I's deliberations on training and performing bodies. As Alex Hutchinson observes in the context of attempts by athletes to lower their body heat with ice-filled vests, reflective sleeves, and ice towels, 'perception is reality'. Although such cooling stratagems do not necessarily change the physiological reality of one's core temperature, they can influence how one *feels* and therefore how one *performs* that reality (Hutchinson 2018: 149). In other words, an important aspect of the work of athletes is to condition their reading (*psychological perception*) of their physical state (*effort ability*) through feeling (*sensorial dimension*). In turn, this process enhances an athlete's psychophysical capacity to strive harder, for longer, and with more *precision*, which, as discussed in the previous chapters, is frequently manifested in the flow–automatization result of repeated practice. As such, the notion of *perception of effort* occupies a central and strategic place in discussions about mind/body relationalities.

Perception of effort foregrounds the role played by feeling. Chapter 3's discussion of pacing in long-distance running and its aesthetic equivalent highlights the subjective variables of *how one feels*. Constructs like Gunnar Borg's Rate of Perceived Exertion (RPE) seek to quantify what is for all intents and purposes an individual's *sense of self* (Chapter 3). And yet the complexity of what constitutes 'feeling' extends beyond an intricate fusion of cognitive and physiological processes. As Matt Fitzgerald articulates it in down-to-earth terms, there is another element at play: 'Perceived effort actually has two layers. The first layer is how the athlete feels. The second layer is how the athlete feels *about* how she feels. The first layer is strictly physiological, whereas the second is emotional, or affective' (Fitzgerald 2016: 48, emphasis in the original). In the context of effort perception, therefore, emotion, or how we feel about how/what we feel, has direct bearing on the quality and outcome of action. This is crucial for athletic and aesthetic performers, especially in the case of actors, dancers, and musicians where the ability to 'touch' audiences (i.e. to *emotionally move* them) is not an optional extra but integral to the communicative aspect of their practice (see

102   *Performer Training for Actors and Athletes*

Introduction). Hence the importance of the question: *What does it mean to 'feel', particularly in the tiered context of 'feeling about how one feels'?*

Fitzgerald's deployment of the word 'feeling' signals two dimensions: the sensorial or 'physiological', *and* the 'emotional'. Reflecting an almost universal trend, Fitzgerald appears to use 'emotional' synonymously with 'affective'. In this multiple echoing of same-words-with-different-meanings and different-words-with-same-meaning, the English language enacts an overlapping complexity that alludes to a variety of related states that include affect, feeling, sensations, emotions, moods, and dispositions. The current chapter recognizes the importance of tracing a path across these phenomena, not so much to fix their meaning (which is impossible due to the ultimately subjective nature of perception and experience), but to enable explorations in theory and practice. Such an exercise provides further insight into the bodyworld of performers, thus complementing the preceding chapters' mind/body perspectives with dimensions of 'feeling'.

I begin with an account of affect to develop an extensive exposition of emotion in terms of constituent components, dynamics, and mechanisms. The discussion, which continues in Chapters 5 and 6 and drives the main thrust of Part II, is illustrated with reference to athletic and aesthetic performance processes.

Affect Theory and Affective Science

The principal terms that are often used in the context of – or even interchangeably with – 'affect' include 'emotion', 'feeling', and 'sensation'. The degree of slippage across these terms can be confusing, depending on the perspective one adopts, and even then, the scope for ambiguity remains. To navigate a way across these overlapping phenomena, a basic outline can be mapped as a point of departure (see Camilleri 2023).

My deployment of these terms is informed by Brian Massumi's reading of French philosopher Gilles Deleuze (1925–1995), especially with reference to the distinction between *affect* and *emotion*. These two phenomena can be placed on a spatio-temporal continuum with *non-conscious* or *preconscious* affect at one end and *conscious* emotion at the other. The middle section of the continuum is populated by sensorial perceptions, i.e. *sensations* of the body in the world (and therefore *of* one's body and *of* the world, which condition one's 'bodyworld' states), and *feelings*, which, as the word implies, can be sensorial (mainly of a tactile nature) and/or emotional (i.e. to have 'feelings' for someone). In other words, here, 'feelings' overlap with 'sensations' and 'emotions', with 'affect' marking a non-conscious relationality between body and world.

Affect, Sensation, Emotion   103

Massumi's conceptualization of affect intersects with an expansive understanding of *movement* (2002: 1–2). For him, affects are 'forces' or 'intensities' between bodies that accompany and shape movement (2002: 15, 24–7). As such, movement marks the continuous stimulation of unformulated relationalities with the material world, some of which surface in our consciousness as the sensations we recognize. Any of these sensations can further evolve into the emotions that, through sociomaterial conditioning, are (re)cognized in specific ways (Massumi 2002: 28; Camilleri 2020a: 27). On this movement-based account of feeling, which aligns well with the action practices of athletic and aesthetic performers, Massumi thus sees sensations and emotions as retrospectively processed readings – what he calls 'back-formations' – of the previously unacknowledged and unrecognized intensity of affects (2002: 7, 10).

To further populate this map of related phenomena, a timeline of occurrence can be based on Eric Shouse's reading of Massumi. Shouse, a cultural studies scholar, packs it in a nutshell thus: 'Feelings are *personal* and *biographical*, emotions are *social*, and affects are *prepersonal*' (2005: online, emphasis in the original). Where does this leave 'sensations'? His definition of feeling as 'a sensation that has been checked against previous experiences and labelled' implies not only that sensation is a kind of feeling but that it occurs *before* feeling. Therefore, in a hypothetical timeline, first there is *sensation* (or sensorial movement), which is then noted and identified as *feeling* (making it 'personal and biographical because every person has a distinct set of previous sensations'), and which is subsequently communicated as *emotion* according to one's socio-cultural conventions and context (Shouse 2005). Crucially, if the emotions of infants are 'direct expressions of affect' because they lack 'language and biography' to experience feelings, affects come prior to all in this multifaceted continuum. In short, this means that *non-conscious sensations* overlap with affects, while *conscious sensations* intersect with feeling. Fine and micro margins, but enough for a working terminology.

The picture of affect presented here belongs to 'affect theory' as distinct from 'affective science'. Although there is diversity within both camps, especially in affect theory as it does not congregate around certain conventions that belong to the 'scientific', their separate genealogies can be sketched thus: 'Writers in affect theory draw on a range of psychological, social, linguistic, and other theories, most often in the service of political analysis. [...] In contrast, affective science has its roots in cognitive science and to a lesser extent social psychology' (Hogan 2016: online). Ruth Leys articulates this distinction as a specific instance of the humanities and sciences divide and of the different protocols and expectations involved (2011: 464–8; see also Papoulias and Callard 2010). Due to their diverse epistemological contexts,

104   *Performer Training for Actors and Athletes*

the terminological picture from affect theory is hardly recognizable from the viewpoint of affective science.

In addition to emotions, feelings, and sensations, affective scientists are interested in the broader picture that includes, amongst other, moods, attitudes, stances, and dispositions, all of which fall under their 'affective' umbrella. For example, contrary to affect theory's privileging of affect as a fundamental non-conscious movement or intensity, Klaus R. Scherer's conceptualization of feeling as a component of – and therefore as distinguishable from – emotion, does not refer to 'affect' at all. Instead, he considers different aspects of feeling in terms of:

(1) 'unconscious reflection and regulation', which includes physiological symptoms, motor expression, action tendencies, and cognitive appraisal;

(2) 'conscious representation and regulation', constituting qualia (the experienced feeling qualities); and

(3) the 'verbalization and communication of emotional experience', i.e. the articulation or 'verbal labelling' of conscious feelings (in Sander and Scherer 2009: 184).

Such a schematic approach to the analysis of emotion, which comes with testable methodologies for each component, is characteristic of affective science, as evidenced, for example, in the extensive entries of *The Oxford Companion to Emotion and the Affective Sciences* (Sander and Scherer 2009). Although affect as understood by an affect theorist subtends and reinforces the phenomena mentioned by Scherer, and although the dynamics of 'labelling' occur in both Shouse (feeling as 'labelled' sensation) and Scherer (emotion as 'labelled' feeling), the variables do not result in quite the same understanding. This is mainly because the 'affective' in affective science is interchangeable with 'emotional' (Hogan 2016), a synonymity that conflicts with much of affect theory since the latter posits crucial differences between the non-conscious and conscious dimensions of emotional states.

Although in this book affect is aligned with Massumi-inspired readings (and therefore with affect theory), the contrasting light cast by affective science is aimed to give volume and dimensionality to the phenomena of feeling. To this end, the *episodic rationalization of emotion* in affective science is adopted for a fuller examination of the diverse facets and characteristics of feeling. This ensures that, for the purposes of analysis, 'affect' and the 'affective' are not left as some kind of homogeneous feeling or integrated experience through the individual-centred selfhood of ipseity.

Rather, Part II's componential concretization of emotion – that is, as *an unfolding episode of different and overlapping occurrences* – foregrounds an appreciation of affect as non-conscious movement that resides in bodies as potential for action.

Experience Emotion Episode

In a pertinent sense, the perception of effort enables an athlete to measure herself against herself, principally through the (sensorial and emotional) *feeling of oneself* and *acting on it*. This relation of one to oneself recalls Massumi's consideration of sensations (the sensorial feeling of movement) in terms of self-referentiality. For him, 'the feeling of having a feeling' that sensations generate amount to a *resonation* – a 'self-continuity' and a 'self-relation' – rather than a subjective split (Massumi 2002: 13–14). On this account, *experience* becomes a way of relating to oneself via sensations and emotions that evolve from affects and which we cultivate as memory in a kind of echo chamber (Camilleri 2020a: 27).

This perspective on experience is highly relevant in the context of a running athlete's perception of effort. It foregrounds the relation of movement to itself, of running to itself due to its continuous and repetitive nature, especially when involving long distances. Moreover, it underlines the double-layered dynamics of sensorial and emotional feeling, and thus of the non-conscious bodyworld intensities in a runner's phenomenological assemblage (Camilleri [2020] 2022: 158–60), e.g. via the equipment or climate/terrain conditions that impact the perception of effort when it comes to pacing.

The case of a runner pacing herself – *against* and *with* herself – magnifies or brings out in sharper relief conditions that exist in other performing bodies, whether that performance is athletic, aesthetic, or daily life. Moreover, the cultivated practice of self-relation that characterizes a runner's training in the perception of effort (e.g. in the monitoring *and* regulating of one's pace as described in Chapter 3), is what marks the *experience* of an 'experienced' athlete. And it is this experience – as *a resonating chamber of feeling* where the 'labelling' of sensations occurs – that constitutes a runner's 'spectrum of intensity' when pacing a run. As Fitzgerald points out: 'Through experience, athletes learn how they *should* feel at various points in a race at a given distance. [...] Any mismatch between how she expects to feel and how she actually feels will cause her to adjust her pace accordingly' (2016: 48, emphasis in the original). This account, which applies not only to runners but to other athletes, aesthetic performers, and individuals more

106   *Performer Training for Actors and Athletes*

broadly, complements Tucker's foregrounding of previous experience in the 'template RPE' (Rate of Perceived Exertion) that, he proposes, contributes to pacing strategy and the regulation of effort during exercise (see Chapter 3; Tucker 2009: 400). Together with one's expectations and knowledge of the task ahead, experience serves to subconsciously monitor and calibrate physiological variables.

With these links to some of the aspects covered in previous chapters, especially with reference to pacing and the role played by experience, it is time to turn attention to matters of feeling via affective science's rationalization of emotion as an episode made up of various phases and elements.

Patrick Colm Hogan, who works primarily at the intersection of literary study with cognitive and affective science, notes that 'we tend to think of emotion as primarily a feeling' (2016: online), which humans experience as individual beings, even when shared by others. However, this is only one aspect – called the 'phenomenological tone' – of what affective scientists denote by 'emotion episode'. Hogan identifies a number of stages and/or states in an emotion episode that can be grouped as follows:

(1) *eliciting conditions*, including aspects from the world-out-there (e.g. climate conditions or world affairs) and from the person herself (e.g. moods, tendencies, character/physiological traits also as informed by social and technical background);
(2) *expressive or communicative outcomes*, which 'spontaneously' transmit the emotion to others and can provoke 'emotion contagion or empathy' (e.g. a cry of fear or tears of sorrow in reaction to an event);
(3) *action readiness*, which primes the 'entire bodily and mental orientation toward behaviour' (e.g. tensing muscles in preparation for a specific action like running away from danger);
(4) *actional outcomes*, consisting of 'the actions themselves' that have already been primed (e.g. running away);
(5) *emotion modulation*, which parallels actional outcomes and marks attempts to 'shift, diminish, sustain, or intensify one's emotional response to a situation' (e.g. lifting one's spirits in a festive occasion despite feeling down);
(6) *cognitive processing*, which can be
    i.   'purely informational' (noting something such as the colour or shape of an object),
    ii. 'positive' or 'top-down' (stressing generalities over particulars),
    iii. 'negative' (stressing particulars over generalities), or
    iv. 'emotion-congruent' (consistent with the current dominant emotion);

Affect, Sensation, Emotion 107

(7) *phenomenological tone*, which signals an 'essentially private [...]
subjective experience that cannot be observed by anyone else or even
phrased in a third-person idiom [...] the one part of emotion that is
ultimately unshareable' (Hogan 2016: online).

Viewing this picture by affective science from the angle of affect theory, it is
possible to trace a hypothetical path that affect follows as it courses from the
body's non-conscious relationality with the world, to the sensations we feel
and the emotions we (re)cognize, to the actions we take.

The various stages in an emotion episode do not follow a linear progression
of discrete stages. Instead, they overlap in the layered space and accelerated
time that recall, respectively, Gregg and Seigworth's 'ever-gathering accretion'
or 'sedimentation' of intensities in bodies (2010: 2–3), and Massumi's speed
of occurrence of these intensities: 'Something that happens too quickly to
have happened, actually, is *virtual*' (2002: 30, emphasis in the original). It
is thus important to bear in mind the layering and speed of the stages in
an emotion episode because this blending of affective science with affect
theory is not intended as a fixed conceptualization but as a framework for
understanding the various facets of feeling. Accordingly, the rest of Part II,
including Chapters 5 and 6, deal with a reading of the constituent elements
in emotion episodes in the light of aesthetic and athletic practices. Such a
reading foregrounds some of the variables that are engaged in all bodies but
which become amplified in overtly somatic practices.

Eliciting Conditions

The first component in an emotion episode that will be re-read here from a
performance viewpoint concerns context. Without going into the potentially
open-ended realms of situational backgrounds and frameworks, one
important feature of *eliciting conditions* incorporates the preparation and
technique training that practitioners undergo to optimize their individual
performance, even in group practices. This includes physical and mental
dexterity as well as related dimensions such as emotional, spiritual, and
other motivational factors that contribute to a body's resilience. Beyond the
boundaries of one's corporeality, and because it is always already a body-in-
the-world, 'eliciting conditions' also refer to the world-out-there.

To illustrate a case of eliciting conditions, one perspective on the bodyworld
engagement of performers involves the use of equipment. Although
the significance of clothes and objects may not be self-evident – they are
often invisible in their ubiquity as part of the visual set-up in performance

108 *Performer Training for Actors and Athletes*

events – they are crucial for somatic practices in mediating felt perception. The sociomateriality of equipment, which includes not only the implications of design and texture to the performing body but also its accessibility (i.e. cost and availability), opens a window on the *eliciting being-in-the-world conditions* of performers. Sports and training clothes and performance costumes delineate one aspect of such equipment.

Organizational and social psychologists Hajo Adam and Adam D. Galinsky coined the term 'enclothed cognition' to describe 'the impact of clothing on the wearer's perceptions and actions', which they see as the incorporation of 'two independent factors – the symbolic meaning of the clothes and the physical experience of wearing them' (2012: 918). This proposal sits well with my formulation of 'habitational action' that, in playing on the etymology of 'habit' as dwelling and as item of clothing, seeks to surpass the embedded dichotomies in compound neologisms like 'bodymind' and 'psychophysical' (Camilleri 2013d: 31) by necessarily bringing together inner action (e.g. memories, emotions) and outer action (e.g. technique, score): 'Since the practitioner is also object and subject of habitation, the act of habitation is necessarily connected to both outer and inner in its occurrence. However, instead of focusing on inner/outer processes, the attention in my investigation is shifted onto the occurrence of the act' (Camilleri 2013a: 162). It was precisely this focus on the *material occurrence* of an act, understood in an expansive manner to include the materiality of context as much as the physicality of the performer, that led to the conceptualization of bodyworld in *Performer Training Reconfigured* (Camilleri 2019). 'Materiality of context' refers to objects, clothes, instruments, and technology as well as the tangible dimensions and implications of socio-cultural behaviour and assumptions, i.e. *socio-cultural affordances* (Christensen and Bicknell 2019: 610–11). In thus combining materiality with psychological and embodiment processes, 'enclothed cognition' marks a specific instance of bodyworld that also applies to athletic and aesthetic performers.

The articulation of bodyworld via the 3As (see Introduction; Camilleri [2020] 2022: 157) sheds light on some of the *contextual conditions* related to equipment in an emotion episode. The gear that athletes wear and deploy as *assemblages* contributes to how they feel (sensorily and emotionally) during exercise and in performance. These feelings can be analysed in terms of the equipment's *affordances* (what they afford the athlete to sense and do). For example, the type of shoe is crucial for runners, whether it is the gel and its placement, or a high stack of lightweight foam that absorbs the impact on the ground, or if carbon plates are also included to propel the body forward for the next step, reducing the effort required and thus maximizing performance.

Runners have different types of shoes for different training and performance situations, e.g. for intervals or speed sessions, steady or tempo

Affect, Sensation, Emotion 109

runs, recovery runs, long runs like marathons, and competitive races, each marking a different 'tool' for specific purposes. However negligible the effect of such affordances may be in an individual step, it accumulates – like Gregg and Seigworth's 'ever-gathering accretion' or 'sedimentation' of intensities in bodies (2010: 2–3) – over the tens of thousands of steps in a marathon. For if there is something wrong with your shoes during a long run, there is something wrong with *you* (e.g. with your feet, legs, balance, perception of heavier effort, feelings of frustration), hence a simple but clear instance of emotional bodyworld states elicited by material conditions. In this regard, Christopher McDougall (2010) and Vybarr Cregan-Reid (2016) make strong cases for barefoot and minimalist running, associating the felt perception that arises from the direct contact with the ground with a different set of affordances involving the world and oneself, the latter including posture and style of running (i.e. forefoot rather than heel strike).

Still within the remit of the 3As, the same equipment can be read in terms of human–non-human *assemblage*, not only the immediate kit–athlete composite on race day but also the human and technology resources (plus infrastructures that enable them) that go into the conception and production of something like a running shoe. Such assemblages are accompanied by all sorts of socio-cultural implications, e.g. the procurement and processing of materials, the sponsorship arrangements that potentially mobilize feelings of prestige and wellbeing, as well as financial security and corporate obligations, all of which come to function as *actants*, i.e. as entities that play a role in the narrative/phenomenology of a specific practice (Camilleri 2019: 39, 92; Camilleri [2020] 2022: 162–4).

Although the psychophysical and/or performance-enhancing value of clothes and objects (including technology) may not be foregrounded or evident in all practices, they can play a role (even a potentially determining one as in the case of footwear in an endurance event), and as such are necessarily entwined with the eliciting conditions of sensations and emotion. Consequently, equipment brings out in higher relief existing conditions and potential variables in *all* practices, including in aesthetic performance as discussed in the following section.

'More Than Just an Actor Dressing'

Bodyworld accretions that function within the broad spectrum of *eliciting conditions* in aesthetic performance can be illustrated in long-term practice with masks, which is an intriguing example that fuses clothing and object. The defamiliarized feeling of one's facial skin as it touches the mask, or of hearing/seeing/smelling oneself through the mask, or even of tasting one's sweat as it accumulates beneath a mask, parallels (and *contributes to*) the effective qualities associated with mask training (Camilleri 2020a: 30–3). As mime teacher Jacques Lecoq states with reference to in-depth engagement with the neutral mask, it allows the actor 'to feel, to touch elementary things with the freshness of beginnings' ([1997] 2002: 38). And this *embodied experience* – which a Massumi-inspired reading of affect would view as *a resonating chamber of feeling* – remains with the actor even when she performs without a mask (Lecoq [1997] 2002: 39). As such, mask work not only *elicits* an actor's sensory conditions but, as is discussed later, also *primes* the actor for more sophisticated emotional layering.

Mask work is not unique in this bodyworld relationality. Similar arguments in the context of aesthetic practices apply with reference to puppetry and object performance (Camilleri [2020] 2022) as well as technology (Camilleri 2019: 67–9; see also Camilleri 2020b regarding the use of gym machines). Less explicit bodyworld accretions that can function as eliciting conditions concern costumes in conventional psychological realist drama. Actors performing in this genre would have a great deal to say about Adam and Galinsky's 'enclothed cognition' concept when the latter ponder:

> Does putting on an expensive suit make people feel more powerful? Does putting on the uniform of a firefighter or police officer make people act more courageously? [...] a seemingly trivial, yet ubiquitous item like an article of *clothing can influence how we think, feel, and act.* Although the saying goes that clothes do not make the man, our results suggest that they do hold a strange power over their wearers.
>
> (Adam and Galinsky 2012: 922, emphasis added)

Considering this book's comparative analysis with athletic practice, we can also add: does putting on the appropriate athletic gear contribute to one's performance? Although one does not 'become' a footballer simply by putting on a football kit, in the context of the appropriate technical training and situation, it does approximate another layer of preparation and engagement of the sort that functions as 'eliciting conditions'. From personal experience, I have come to discover (sometimes at the cost of aching muscles, sore nipples, broken toenails, and blisters) that wearing the appropriate gear for endurance running is not merely a superficial or cosmetic extra but has functional needs.

Moreover, even the act of preparing one's clothing and equipment on the eve of an important run functions as a quasi-meditational ritual that completes the psychophysical training and transforms one into a 'runner'. Just

Affect, Sensation, Emotion   111

as an actor does not 'become' a judge, a priest, or a queen merely by wearing their costume, but is a reflection in body (apparel) and mind (psychology) that *completes* the work of building that character, so can the appropriate athletic gear condition 'how we think, feel and act'. In Stanislavski's words, as expressed by the fictional assistant director Ivan Rakhmanov:

> 'When you've played just one role, it will be clear to you just what a wig, a beard, a costume, a prop means to you and how much you need it for the character you're playing.
>
> 'Only someone who has gone down the long, difficult road of not only looking for the soul but the bodily form of a human being/role that has formed in their imagination and then taken shape in their own body, can understand what every feature, detail, object connected with the being they have to bring alive means. [...]
>
> 'A costume or a prop we have found for a character cease to be mere objects and become holy relics. [...] This is *more than just an actor dressing.* This the moment when he puts on his *robes* [original emphasis]. It is *a very important, psychological moment.* That is why you can tell real artists by the way they relate to their costume and hand props, the way they love and care for them.'
>
> (Stanislavski 2008: 575, emphasis added)

It is precisely that 'psychological moment', as stimulated by the senses and developed in training, that underscores the conditions for the subsequent enactment of emotions in aesthetic performance.

Expressive or Communicative Outcomes

The second component in an emotion episode that Hogan identifies deals with *expressive or communicative outcomes*, which consists of unplanned somatic reactions that 'do not serve directly to alter or maintain the situation [but] to convey the emotion to those present' (Hogan 2016). Possible equivalents in athletic practice are the cries (or 'grunts') of tennis players when hitting forcefully a ball with a racket or the heavy breathing (even bordering on hyperventilating) when running, especially uphill with speed at maximum effort.

The relatively incipient and shapeless quality of this component places it close to the relational intensities of affect in that its 'spontaneity' and formlessness can be compared to Shouse's account of an infant's reactive

112   *Performer Training for Actors and Athletes*

'direct expressions of affect' (2005). Such a comparison needs to be made with caution, especially in the case of a tennis player's grunts that can hardly be either spontaneous or non-conscious. Unlike Shouse's infants, as an adult and as a trained practitioner, the athlete possesses ample 'language and biography' for the non-conscious intensity of affects to emerge uninhibited (psychologically), unhindered (physically), and therefore unformed (behaviourally). Indeed, the eruption of grunts or breathing sounds can be part of an athlete's preparation and technical training to optimize her performance (e.g. to power a volley shot or contain an accelerating heart rate) as well as to make the most of the situation (e.g. grunting as a tactic to irritate, distract, mislead, or otherwise disrupt the competitor, including via emotion contagion to condition others to experience the outcome/feeling as their own).

Notwithstanding the above caveats, expressive outcomes have particular significance due to their relative proximity to affect when compared to other stages in an emotion episode. Especially pertinent in the context of aesthetic performance and its fundamental distinction from athletic practice (i.e. its *communicative* rather than competitive agenda), are the 'communicative outcomes' that Hogan notes in film and theatre through the 'emotional mirroring' of audiences. Such mirroring occurs due to an 'overlap between the neurologically based systems that respond to one's observation of other people's behaviours and the systems involved in one's own enactment of related behaviours (e.g. other people's smiling and one's own smiling)' (Hogan 2016). If Hogan is correct, expressive outcomes resonate with some kind of primordial capacity or survival mechanism that resides as a trace in human beings.

Affective and cognitive scientist Giovanna Colombetti (2014) has proposed the concept of 'primordial affectivity' to emphasize that sense-making activity is not only marked by *cognition* (as in the enactive approach) but is 'simultaneously also *affective*'. That is, communication at its most basic level and as automatic expression – let alone at the sophisticated heights of aesthetic performance – involves 'feelings': 'Affectivity thus characterized is not just broader but "deeper" than the emotions and moods of affective science, in the sense that it grounds them or makes them possible; in other words, without the primordial capacity to be affected, no specific emotions and moods would appear' (Colombetti 2014: 2). Colombetti's view of affectivity, which can be located somewhere between the emotional states of affective science and the preconscious relationality of affect theory, is not dependent on the nervous system in isolation but is enacted by the organism as a whole at the same time as it brings forth a world of significance (2014: 21). This combination of sense (perception) and sense-making (meaning), however

Affect, Sensation, Emotion 113

primitive and latent, also informs the mirroring that Hogan aligns with the expressive outcomes of aesthetic performance.

Another aspect that emerges from Hogan's point concerns the *speed* of that mirroring and the implications to consciousness. In adults – and therefore including athletes, actors, and other performers – the emotional mirroring that is associated with communicative outcomes occurs too fast ('spontaneously') to be consciously controlled by the audience. That is, by the time we realize what happened or is happening (e.g. feelings of sadness or relief), the affective exchange would have occurred. This speed of occurrence recalls what Massumi understands by 'virtual' when he describes affects as '*virtual synesthetic perspectives*' (Massumi 2002: 35), that is, 'that affects happen so quickly that we register them only *after* the event as sensations, emotions, and other experiential qualities' (Camilleri 2019: 151). On this account, a 'spontaneous' cry of fear, although not quite as 'virtual' and despite speaking the 'language' of other cries of fear uttered before it, comes closest to affect's unformed expression. The grunt of a tennis player while volleying or of a boxer when striking a punch, or a runner's vocalized breathing, no doubt *forms* part of their training, and therefore *forms* their embodiment, thus qualifying their 'spontaneity'. However, they can still be aligned with affect's 'virtuality' of sensory occurrence by coinciding with the *dynamic*, rather than the *content*, of that release in performing bodies.

Stage Fright

The uncontrollable experience of 'stage fright' in aesthetic performance, which parallels 'choking' in athletic practice (see Chapter 2; Fitzgerald 2016: 86–99; Cappuccio et al. 2019: 111–13), provides some insight into a specific set of expressive or communicative outcomes. The discussion on stage fright by theatre scholar Nicholas Ridout begins with an analysis of an incident between the two imaginary interlocutors in Stanislavski's *An Actor Prepares* ([1936] 1989), i.e. the experienced director Arkady Tortsov and the young acting student Konstantin Nazvanov better known as Kostya. Ridout picks up on the 'something somatic as much or as well as psychological' aspects of Kostya's 'new unexpected sensations [that] surged inside' him (Stanislavski [1936] 1989: 8) when rehearsing on stage for the first time (Ridout 2006: 36). These sensations were amplified on performance night in front of an audience: 'My throat became constricted, my sounds all seemed to go to a high note. My hands, feet, gestures and speech all became violent, I was ashamed of every word, of every gesture. I blushed, clenched my hands, and pressed myself against the back of the armchair' (Stanislavski [1936] 1989: 11). In

114   *Performer Training for Actors and Athletes*

other words, despite his preparations, Kostya could not control his body, let alone express the feelings of Othello, the character he was interpreting (cf. Aquilina 2013: 232). Kostya's experience recalls the paralysing internal focus of attention and the self-consciousness of choking in sports (see Chapter 2 and Moran 2012: 88).

And yet, Kostya was communicating 'something somatic [and] psychological' despite his intentions and volition: his body was, literally in a physiological sense, *acting up*. Ridout's explanation is revealing in the context of the current chapter when he observes that Kostya 'is being robbed of his adulthood, forced into an immobile, helpless, squeaky state of being: *a state of infancy*' (2006: 38, emphasis added). Such a 'state of infancy' parallels Kostya's inexperience – or lack of resonance in his echo chamber of feelings – as an actor. Kostya does not know what it *feels* – indeed what it *means* – to act on stage in front of an audience. He does not have any prior *experience* (or the aesthetic equivalent of an athlete's 'template RPE') against which to compare these 'surging sensations', to re*cognize* them and channel them to his own ends as the 'knowing' Tortsov does (2006: 35). As such, this aspect of the novice actor can be viewed in the light of Shouse's 'direct expressions of affect' by infants who lack 'a history of previous experiences from which to draw in assessing the continuous flow of sensations coursing through his or her body' (2005: online).

Ridout acknowledges the significance of Kostya's experience, situated as it is in the very first chapter of Stanislavski's *An Actor Prepares*: 'At the very start of the elaboration of his famous system – still the most substantial and influential source for actor-training in the West – Stanislavski makes stage fright the precondition of theatrical success' (Ridout 2006: 40). On this account, therefore, the phenomenon of stage fright, including the expressive and communicative outcomes of its physiological *and* emotional dimensions, is linked with processes of emergence and development, which can be both positive, like Kostya's growth as an actor, or debilitating, if it becomes recurrent. Of course, stage fright is not exclusive to novice performers because variations of it (like unexpectedly going blank and forgetting lines) can afflict experienced performers, including athletes choking in high pressure situations. However, its causes and effects are magnified in novices, making it clearer for exemplification purposes.

The differentiating factor between expressive/communicative outcomes and other stages in an emotion episode concerns whether or not the event directly impacts the situation by altering or maintaining it: communicative outcomes like cries of fear or the uncontrollable behaviour of stage fright *convey* the event/emotion to others. Albeit a 'doing' in its own right, a communicative outcome often functions as a *comment on* rather than as a

Affect, Sensation, Emotion 115

stimulus for action, thus leading straight to its *cognitive processing* stage (e.g. realizing what just happened). If, on the other hand, that cry of fear alters or maintains the situation, for example by running away or by resolutely standing one's ground, or like Kostya's transformation of his rage for his 'helpless infancy' into the rage of Othello (Ridout 2006: 39), then it leads to *action readiness* and *actional outcome*.

Action Readiness

Action readiness is what a 'training of affect' would aspire to achieve in psychosomatic practices ... if only it were possible. 'Priming' is a better word than 'training' as one cannot operate directly on non-conscious affect. An alternative option to an impossible direct training on affect is to intervene at the level of 'eliciting conditions' in a way that brings about 'autonomous' action that simultaneously also enables its 'readiness'. *Autonomous* (as distinct from 'automatic') action can be aligned with the corporeal dispositions that emerge (seep or erupt) when prompted by the material conditions of a situation (Camilleri 2020a: 27–8; see also Camilleri 2018a: 36–40). These dispositions reside as 'ever-gathering accretion' in bodies (Gregg and Seigworth 2010: 2–3) that accumulate from the multitude of unacknowledged and unrecognized intensities of affects (Massumi 2002: 7, 10). Such phenomena of 'the body taking action on its own – a re-acting to the situation without explicit consciousness' (Camilleri 2020a: 28) can be associated with John-David Dewsbury's 'affective habit ecologies' from affect theory and human geography, which refer to the impact of place on human behaviour (Dewsbury 2012). They can be also compared with J. Kevin O'Regan and Alva Noë's 'sensorimotor contingencies' from enactive cognition, which link movement and sensory stimulation in the background of consciousness and which vary according to a changing situation (O'Regan and Noë 2001, see Chapter 1).

Since corporeal dispositions are emergent from the material *conditions* of an occurrence, and as such can be affiliated with bodyworld *affordances*, one way of illustrating them is through what in the science and psychology of sports deals with the broader repertoires of *real game situations*. Game strategies of this kind emphasize 'bodily dispositions and affordances in the environment' that condition the 'habitual interactions and affective patterns, which constitute the cognitive agent's [the athlete's] structural coupling with real-world scenarios' (Cappuccio 2019: xix).

It is important to clarify that 'autonomous dispositions' are not the same as the automatic actional patterns that result from drill-based activities – e.g.

kicking a ball over and over again in the same manner – but to action tendencies that accumulate with experience from free play and in real-world situations – e.g. kicking a ball while playing a game, i.e. while running, turning, or falling, or trying to avoid an opponent, or to score or pass it to a colleague, or on a dubious section of turf, or while it is raining, hot, or windy, or during the day or under floodlights, or when losing and time is running out, etc., and myriad combinations of all these (see Ford and O'Connor 2019). Consequently, it is justifiable to distinguish between automatic and autonomous action. As surveyed in the Introduction, the *Handbook of Embodied Cognition and Sport Psychology* (Cappuccio 2019) has an entire section dedicated to 'Affordances and Action Selection' that examines and exemplifies such real-world conditions and strategies (2019: 535–621), all of which highlight 'the reciprocal coupling between skillful embodied agents, with their sensorimotor predispositions, and the environmental contingencies that solicit them' (Cappuccio 2019: xxix).

Although this is *not* affect training (because the moment 'affect' is identified as such, let alone worked upon, it becomes something else, *a back-formation*), it unavoidably operates – by multiplication and expansion – on the incipient tendencies that accumulate below the level of consciousness from the unformulated relationalities that the body ceaselessly generates with the world around. In other words, while not selecting (i.e. retrospectively forming) affects from the available options, *priming practices* like extensive real-world game experience re-*place* (by repositioning to the background or foreground) or overwhelm (by the sheer quantity available due to the time dedicated to the activity) certain relational intensities and not others. Since this does not work *directly on* but *around* behaviour, 'priming' is indeed a more accurate term than 'training'.

'Priming' *readies* the performing body, it *makes* the body physiologically *ready*, orienting it towards (rather than resulting in) specific behavioural traits, for example, it tenses the relevant muscles in preparation for a specific action. And the status of that priming of muscular tension is often autonomous and dispositional, i.e. not always conscious (e.g. we do not think of flexing the relevant facial muscles before we smile). On the other hand, 'training' (which entails the back-formation of certain activities, and therefore involves exercises and technique) is more directly associated with *actional outcomes* and as such pertains to the subsequent component in an emotion episode. Before proceeding to discuss *actional outcomes* in Chapter 5, the current exposition concludes with a possible equivalent in aesthetic performance of the bodily dispositions marked by *action readiness*, specifically as it resonates with real-world scenarios in sports.

Affect, Sensation, Emotion 117

Improvisation and Real-World Play

Although aesthetic performances are relatively fixed in score or choreographic structure when compared to the free flow of competitive sports events (see Chapter 3), improvisation sessions in the performing arts share some common ground with real-world situations in sports. Both improvisatory and real-world practices can be viewed as *preparatory* or *formative* activities rather than as prescribed 'technique training'. As theatre practitioner and scholar Simon Murray observes: 'Compared to the more circumscribed word "training", *preparation* seems to imply a process of getting ready, of open-endedness and an unwillingness to close down on possible options and choices' (Murray 2003: 64, emphasis in the original). At the same time, improvisation and real-world conditions are *finishing* practices that encapsulate performance in its entirety, with a beginning, middle, and end, as well as the modulations and exigencies that come with open (i.e. not predetermined) itineraries. In both instances, the individual (and the collective) is freer to *play* compared to public performances and competitions.

It is precisely this opportunity to *play* that can be seen to nurture the priming capacity associated with *action readiness*. The Introduction acknowledged the dynamics of play and its implications for action, both *within* somatic practices like theatre and sports but also *beyond* in terms of the frame of mind it affords. It can be problematic to pin down exactly what 'play' comprises for it is not a specific thing to do (a *what*). And although it is related to *how* one does, it is not even a manner or style. Play can be viewed as a kind of 'inhabiting something' since one always '*plays with* something' – in the context of theatre this involves objects, clothes, masks, text, other performers, imaginary equivalents of all these (including a made-up language), and almost anything else. To better understand the phenomenon, it is useful to consider it in the context of a practice.

Although play and improvisation feature in the work of many performance-makers, it is closely identified with Lecoq whose specific understanding of *le jeu* ('play' or 'playfulness') he developed from *commedia dell'arte*, Jacques Copeau (1879–1949), and other sources (Murray 2003: 10–13, 29–33). As a fundamental priming capacity for movement, Lecoq's *le jeu* is particularly pertinent to this volume because, as Mark Evans observes: 'The notion of play lies not just at the heart of Lecoq's ideas about theatre, but is also central to his understanding of sport' (2012a: 168) and as such intersects the processes of actors and athletes. Lecoq's interest in movement, from his early experiences in sports to his later and deeper pursuit in physical acting, makes

118   *Performer Training for Actors and Athletes*

his work even more relevant in a discussion on emotion episodes informed by Massumi's reading of *affect as movement* (Camilleri 2019: 166–7).

Lecoq's play comprises sheer delight and resourcefulness, but not only that. In his world, *le jeu* is accompanied by what he calls *disponibilité* (availability, openness) and *complicité* (involvement, togetherness), all three marking key elements in improvisation aimed at fostering expressive potential that a mastery of technique alone does not guarantee. Again, we are faced with 'potential' (which is always *incipient*) that is linked with a capacity of doing (a *readiness*) rather than with a content or form of doing.

Drilling deeper, Murray unpacks Lecoq's understanding of play as follows:

> Being 'aware of the theatrical dimension' removes play or playfulness from mere pleasurable self-indulgence and provides it with *context and purpose*. To 'shape an improvisation' suggests territory where the actor has a degree of physical, vocal and spatial freedom to be *inventive*, rather than being merely a conduit for the director or playwright. [...] Without play – in its richest and most nuanced form – spectators will never be properly engaged in the theatrical event.
>
> (Murray 2003: 65, emphasis added)

From this angle, then, playfulness for Lecoq is neither a self-centred activity nor structureless freedom but an all-encompassing experience for player *and* beholder. For the player, because she is immersed in her playing, and therefore following some kind of logic. Even when *not* predetermined like that of a play-text, this 'logic' emerges *during* the work and is acknowledged retrospectively as a *back-formation* (see Chapter 6). For the beholder, because she is engaged by the movement (the 'life' or 'living structure' according to Lecoq [1997] 2002: 20) of the player's doing.

How does such an appreciation of 'playfulness' compare with what happens in sports when 'playing' a game? Except for activities like certain track and field disciplines that depend on specific embodied patterns, many forms of sports involve an improvisation of sorts. For instance, every football or tennis match is unlike any other because the variables at play render the development and outcome of the event unique. This is unlike a theatre or dance performance with blocked vocal/physical scores that, however open to subtle changes and variations, follow the same predetermined structure. Nevertheless, the 'freedom' of play in football or tennis – even in the game scenarios of practice matches – is still qualified by the rules and procedures that regulate the discipline, e.g. a footballer cannot score a goal using her hands.

Affect, Sensation, Emotion   119

Although there are different types of improvisation in aesthetic performance, including within time-based, space-restricted, and movement-tasked structures that resemble typical sports activity, free play in theatre, dance, and performance training processes has the potential to 'play around' even with the rules. In aesthetic performance, it can be possible to have the football equivalent of scoring a goal with a hand.

These overlapping differences between aesthetic and sport practices demand a nuanced distinction between play and games. Tim Etchells, artistic director of Forced Entertainment, sheds some light on the matter: 'Play is looser than games – it has a chameleon-like, mutable quality. It allows a shift of rules, a shift between different positions – an "I can change *the paradigm* we are working in" quality' (cited in Murray 2003: 67, emphasis added). Of course, the improvising performer does abide by certain rules, mainly, but not exclusively, societal such as not harming others or damaging property. However, she is distinctly freer than the athlete to ignore the rules of the 'paradigm'. Or rather, to *make up* the rules as she 'plays around'.

In aesthetic performance contexts, including those inspired by Lecoq, improvisation does not only involve *dynamics of play* (i.e. *within* a structure) but also the *mechanisms and strategies of play* (i.e. *with* structure). Like Jean-François Lyotard's postmodern artist (1984: 81), the improvising performer works without rules but *towards* them, even if those rules are recognized retrospectively, *after* the event, and eventually discarded at the end of a session. Crucially for an understanding of *action readiness* in an emotion episode, it is precisely the *residue* of that discarding – what in Massumi are the incipient intensities not taken up but which reside as potential or dormant tendencies – that has value in such activity.

As Etchells continues: 'Play is a state in which meaning is flux, in which possibility thrives, in which versions multiply' (in Murray 2003: 67). For what play 'teaches' is not a content, a technique, or an aesthetic, but *corporeal dispositions*, i.e. ways of inhabiting an event, be that aesthetic, sports, or daily life. As such, play marks a *dispositional or attitudinal readiness* that 'accretes' physiological and mental ways of being, and which in turn 'secretes' (seeps, erupts, or otherwise prompts or conditions) behaviour in particular situations. In both the Introduction and Conclusion, this understanding of play (in combination with a collaborative competitiveness and self-organizing pacing) is associated with a modality of performing and behaving I identify as '*via athletae*'.

With behaviour we arrive at *actional outcomes*, the stage at the crossroads of Hogan's formulation of emotion episodes. In more ways than one, this is *the* main action event of aesthetic, athletic, and daily performers. All previous stages, from *eliciting conditions* to *expressive/communicative outcomes* and *action readiness*, lead up to actional outcomes. Conversely, all subsequent stages are based on it, from *emotion modulation* to *cognitive processing* and *phenomenological tone*. Accordingly, Chapter 5 focuses on the actional dimensions of emotional experience in performance.

5

Performing Feeling:
Action, Intention, Transformation

This chapter looks at *the emotional dimension of action* in aesthetic and athletic performance and at its implications for performer training. To this end, it adopts from the preceding chapter a hybrid methodological approach that combines insights from affect theory and affective science. The bringing together of these two perspectives, whose terminological differences reflect deeper epistemological divergences (see Chapter 4), is intentionally aimed at shedding intersectional light on what is often an elusive topic.

The consideration from affective science of a series of overlapping stages in an emotion episode compels the understanding of affective states as the fundamental phenomenon from which physical action emerges. Meanwhile, affect theory's emphasis on sensorial and emotional feeling, especially its explanation of *movement* as incipient and actualized potential in body–world relationalities, provides details at micro levels and connects what risks becoming a compartmentalized rationalization of an essentially organic flow.

Affective science approximates Stanislavski-based practices of contemplating character and plot development as an event that pre-dates the present to include factors and experiences that lead to the current situation. That this perspective belongs to a psychological realist aesthetic is no coincidence considering its close study of human behaviour in daily life. For other aesthetics like physical theatre and dance that do not necessarily involve daily behavioural patterns or logic, a more rewarding starting point for analysis is movement. Physical action – or the behavioural design of bodies in the here and now – is what audiences see on stage and what first conditions their reading before any emotional messaging or interpretation. It is thus in this regard that a focus on the episodic nature of emotions serves as a material deconstruction of action by foregrounding the *contexts* that give rise to it and the *adjustments* that subsequently shape it.

Chapter 4 dealt with the 'contextual' aspects of emotion episodes as presented in Patrick Colm Hogan's (2016) account from affective science, i.e. *eliciting conditions*, *expressive/communicative outcomes*, and *action readiness*. The present chapter focuses on the *actional outcome* of these components

122   *Performer Training for Actors and Athletes*

as well as on one of its subsequent 'adjustments', *emotion modulation*. Chapter 6 discusses two other adjustments or qualities of actional outcomes: *cognitive processing* and *phenomenological tonality*. It is important to reiterate the point made in the previous chapter that these components are neither discrete nor always linearly sequential, and that they often overlap and occur at accelerated times, especially in moments of transition that reinforce the experiential continuity and integrity of the event.

The 'adjustment' components of actional outcomes (i.e. emotion modulation, cognitive processing, and phenomenological tone) also involve the attentional, physiological, and other monitoring and regulatory processes discussed in Chapters 1, 2, and 3. For instance, Samuele Marcora's psychobiological model of perceived effort, explained in Chapter 3, exemplifies such ongoing intra-relationality between actional outcome and adjustment processes by positing that athletic activity is influenced by how one (emotionally) *feels* about (physiological and sensorial) *feeling*.

As can be seen in this seven-part conceptualization of emotion episodes, the central or crossroads component is occupied by the *actional outcome* performed by the individual. This is the action and behaviour that spectators see in a theatre, sports arena, or daily life. Its halfway placement on this episode-continuum of emotion implies that, despite its evident foregrounding in execution and reception, it is neither the starting point nor the destination of a process, hence this chapter's consideration of action in the light of what precedes and follows it.

From Action Readiness to Actional Outcomes

Actional outcomes are necessarily related to *action readiness* in that they are the actualized manifestation of the same process. Although not every 'readiness' leads to a fully fledged 'outcome', all outcomes are 'readied' in one way or other. Hogan explains the 'priming' of action readiness as 'the partial activation of [motor] routines, below the threshold of enactment', qualifying it as 'the preparatory tensing or relaxation of the musculature, and other, relevant physiological orientations' (2016). On this account, therefore, the difference between action *readiness* and *outcome* is limited and fulfilled enactment respectively, e.g. between the tensing of muscles to kick a ball and kicking it. To drill deeper into this distinction, reference can be made to a type of exercise that is used in sports and that has been adapted by a theatre practice to research the nature of physical actions in performance.

Hogan's distinction between the partial activation and the full enactment of an action recalls *isometry*, a type of physical exercise where no movement

Action, Intention, Transformation

is apparent despite engaging a set of muscles. 'Isometry' was a new approach to sports training developed in the mid-twentieth century. As its etymology suggests (Greek *isos* 'equal' plus *metron* 'measure'), it involves the static contraction of a muscle without any visible movement in the angle of the joint. Instead of lifting weights or using similar equipment to enhance the muscular capability of athletes, isomeric pushes or pulls function by generating and maintaining an opposite but equal force in different parts of the body. An example of an isometric task is the 'plank', which stimulates the body's core musculature while holding still for as long as possible a position similar to a push-up. Other examples include pressing the palms together in front of the torso and pushing against a door frame. In such exercises, maximal contraction of the muscle is needed whilst remaining static. The dynamics of this kind of exercise parallel the muscular activation of *action readiness* in an emotion episode.

The implications of isometry for human behaviour, especially for bodies in performance, can be far-reaching, as evidenced in the work of Ingemar Lindh and his theatre group the Institutet för Scenkonst:

The isometric approach developed by the Institute involved the isolation of the instant immediately preceding the most dynamic moment of a specific action – for example, the moment before contact when kicking a ball. Later, the focus shifted to stops at any point in mid-action which are then completed *without having to generate a new impulse*. In these cases it is necessary to retain intensity in the stillness in order to ensure that the continuation of a particular action is not a new beginning. In the stops thus generated: 'The action [had to] be continued mentally' ([Lindh 2010: 25]). By pushing the investigation to extreme consequences, a number of discoveries were made, including the fundamental difference between (physical) impulse and (mental) intention. The continuation announced by an isometric stop in the shift of intention from a physical to a mental plane [...] marked an integral aspect of mental precision.

(Camilleri 2008b: 436, emphasis in the original)

'Mental precision' refers to specific terminology employed by the Institutet to mark the movement or *action in the mind* that precedes its physical manifestation. It played a crucial role in Lindh's research on collective improvisation as performance, which eschewed directorial montage and fixed scores, foregrounding instead the performers' relational work with their material, each other, and the 'social situation' of the performance (Camilleri 2008a: 84–6).

124   *Performer Training for Actors and Athletes*

'Mental precision' does not entail a predominance of mind over body because, in their work, the Institutet considered 'mental action' or 'action in the mind' as a physical phenomenon (i.e. as an integral part of physical action) via *intention*:

> In Lindh's research, mental precision is related to 'intention', which, in the Institutet's vocabulary, is a composite of 'to tend toward' (to project and place oneself in the direction of) and 'tension' (to mobilize one's energy in a specific direction). Intention thus understood refers to the movement of the mind at the beginning of every act and indicates an act's mental direction, which can be concretized both through stillness (non-movement) and movement.
>
> (Camilleri 2011: 304)

This example from the performing arts about practical research on isometry within the context of specific psychosomatic projection chimes with the 'entire bodily and mental orientation toward behaviour' that characterizes *action readiness* in Hogan's account. It also concretizes – by *problematizing* – the relational distinction between *action readiness* and *outcomes*.

The notion of 'action in the mind' and intentionality is of crucial importance in theatre processes, especially in the twentieth-century context of Konstantin Stanislavski's psychological realism and of subsequent developments like Jerzy Grotowski's more physical aesthetic and twenty-first-century performances like Katie Mitchell's that combine Stanislavski and Grotowski influences (Shevtsova and Innes 2009: 180–2; Rebellato 2010: 324, 327). If the first three chapters of this book have told us anything from the perspective of athletic activity and sports science, it is that intentionality in physical action is not always *entirely* or *consciously* intentional. That is, elite-level training in sports is often aimed at degrees of automaticity where actional precision is achieved 'without thinking about it', for too much self-awareness and internal focus leads to the self-consciousness of choking or to missing the opportunity due to the evolving circumstances of play (see Chapter 2).

On the other hand, doing something 'without thinking about it' does not necessarily exclude intentionality on a broader metacognitive level, just as we saw with pacing in Chapter 3. For example, an attacking footballer's intention is to score a goal. This applies even when she does not think about how, where, and when she kicks the ball but reacts to the affordances of a given situation that, in any case, she had helped bring about by her tactical reading of the game. As discussed in Chapter 2 with reference to the 'paradox of control' in optimal flow experiences, 'one has a sense of exercising control

Action, Intention, Transformation

without trying to be in control' (Jackson 1996: 77). In the present context, this paradoxical kind of 'control' applies to or can be aligned with the 'action in the mind' and 'mental precision' of intentionality in aesthetic performance, i.e. as an embodied state of mind that treads a fine line between activation and release. To explore *actional outcomes* in emotion episodes and in other circumstances, the following sections delve deeper into the liminal space that isometry inhabits between readiness and outcome, priming and activation, partial and full enactment.

Thought-Action

In isometric activity, action readiness coincides with – *is* – the actional outcome, thus suggesting a 'snapshot freeze' of a psychophysical intention. This *actional pause* (i.e. a pause that is an action) allows the phenomenon to be studied in a manner that slows down – just as it magnifies – what occurs at 'virtual' speed in the affective process (see Chapter 4). However, this is only half of the story in the Institutet's case because in their adaptation of isometry, the halted action is continued 'mentally', e.g. the bodymind intention/act of kicking proceeds on a mental level, it is 'only' the physical manifestation that changes. The objective is to imbue the actional outcome of that stop with a liveness (precisely an *action readiness*) that can be aligned with what Lindh's corporeal mime teacher, Étienne Decroux, called 'active immobility' or 'mobile immobility' (Decroux [1963] 1985: 51).

Eugenio Barba considers 'active immobility' as a general principle that occurs in somatic practices across different cultural milieus, be they aesthetic, athletic, artisan, or in daily life ([1993] 1995: 55–6). He uses the Norwegian word for impulse, *sats*, to characterize a particular aspect of embodied technical know-how:

> The dancing feet of a soccer player, and the fantasy of *sats* – of impulses – of a handball player who, hovering in the air, manages to surprise opponents who jump in front of him/her [...]; a carpenter's way of planing, the hammer blows of the blacksmith who forges a glowing piece of iron, the rhythmic accuracy of the mason marrying one brick to another [...], the powerful behaviour of an actor/dancer who intensifies the life of the stage reality: all this is technique learned through a long apprenticeship. It is know-how guided by experience and principles [...]. They are *methods*, ways of proceeding that lead towards the effectiveness of an intention.
>
> (Barba 2021: 223, emphasis in the original)

126 *Performer Training for Actors and Athletes*

Barba's list exemplifies a broad spectrum of actional outcomes, all of which involve *sats* as a fundamental principle in his understanding of theatre anthropology (Barba and Savarese 2006).

In a section entitled '*Sats* – the energy can be suspended' in *The Paper Canoe* ([1993] 1995: 54–9), Barba identifies the phenomenon in a number of aesthetic performance traditions in history and across cultures (cf. Grotowski 2006: 268). In addition to Decroux's 'mobile immobility', Barba's exposition ranges from Vsevolod Meyerhold's *predigra* ('pre-acting') as a moment of tension that leads to action, to Grotowski's 'kind of silence before the movement' that 'can occur as a stop of the action' (Barba [1993] 1995: 55), from the transitional *tangkis* between one posture, direction, or level to another in Balinese dance theatre (57), to the *liang xiang* stops in positions of precarious balance in Peking Opera (57), as well as the tensed stops or stillness of *io-in* in Japanese Noh theatre (58). Barba even makes a case that Stanislavski's practical understanding of *rhythm* can be aligned with *sats* in instances such as when the Russian director asks his actors to 'stand [still] in the correct rhythm' (58–9; cf. Barba and Savarese 2006: 92).

In some of these instances, the caesura of the impulse is minimal but still perceptible, such as a carpenter's repetitive action when using a hand wood planer to smoothen surfaces but which she can halt at any time. In other instances, it is perceptible only on a kinaesthetic level, e.g. in a succession of continuous but sudden changes of direction as a footballer attempts to dribble a ball past opponents by misleading their readings of her intention (cf. Barba 2010: 91). And in other situations, it can be more pronounced and extended, such as in a mime performance. Even in the latter case, where 'staccato movement' is an essential part of the aesthetic (Decroux [1963] 1985: 51), this does not entail motion by fits and starts, for 'if the *sats* are too marked, they become inorganic' (Barba [1993] 1995: 56). The performance of an experienced mime is not punctured by the kind of stops that reflect a rupture between intention/thought and action – a rupture caused by a lack of control due to insufficient technique and know-how. Rather, a mime etude of the type envisaged by Decroux is punctuated by stops that, in the continuity of their corporeal *mobile* immobility, give shape and texture – and therefore *meaning* – to the movement. It was precisely this continuity that Lindh explored and developed as 'mental precision' in the application of the isometric principle from sports training to his theatre practice.

The pregnant pause of *sats* – 'pregnant' because the psychophysical energy/ action is 'conceived' in its *readiness* but not yet 'delivered' as *outcome* – can be located in what Barba calls the 'structure of *sats*', i.e. in the space and time between impulse and counter-impulse (2010: 57): 'the instant which precedes the action, when all the energy is already there, ready to intervene,

Action, Intention, Transformation 127

but as if suspended' (Barba [1993] 1995: 39). This liminal aspect of *sats* is also manifested in what can be called its 'anatomy', i.e. the stance that makes it possible:

> [Odin Teatret] actors tend to assume a *position* in which the knees, very slightly bent, contain the *sats,* the impulse towards *an action which is as yet unknown and which can go in any direction*: to jump or crouch, step back or to one side, to lift a weight. The *sats* is the basic *posture* found in sports – in tennis, badminton, boxing, fencing – when you need to be ready to react.
>
> (Barba [1993] 1995: 5–6, emphasis added)

Slightly bent knees mean that the legs are not blocked, that the individual does not need to un(b)lock her psychophysical resources: the door is open, and the resources are 'all-ready' (i.e. *already* mobilized in immobility), and what remains is the decision/impulse, the *intention*, to move in space/time.

The embodied liminality of *sats* also marks the aspect that has preoccupied the first three chapters of this book: the relation between thought and action. Very tellingly, one of the ways that Barba refers to *sats* in *The Paper Canoe* is by the term 'thought-action' because it eliminates the split between thought and physical action. Specifically, he describes *sats* as 'a minute charge with which *the thought innervates the action* and is experienced as *thought-action,* energy, rhythm in space' ([1993] 1995: 57, emphasis added):

> The *sats* is the moment in which the action is *thought/acted by the entire organism* [...]. It is the point at which one decides to act. [...] It is the tightening or the gathering together of oneself from which the action departs. It is [...] [a]n athlete, a tennis player or boxer, immobile or moving, ready to react. It is John Wayne facing an adversary. It is Buster Keaton about to take a step. It is Maria Callas on the verge of an aria.
>
> (Barba [1993] 1995: 54–5, emphasis added)

The shift from *readiness* to *outcome* in all these actions, which very relevantly range from sports to the performing arts, therefore, is a thought-action that necessarily overlaps with intentionality.

Barba's reference to the role played by the nervous system in thought-action processes is revealing, irrespective of whether his deployment of the term 'innervates' is quasi-metaphorical rather than scientific. As expounded in Chapter 3, Tim Noakes's 'central governor' theory holds that in endurance activities the central nervous system reduces the neural activation of muscle fibres to regulate the body's performance to maintain physical and chemical

128   *Performer Training for Actors and Athletes*

stability (homeostasis). According to Noakes, the central governor does not function entirely on a voluntary level and can even override explicit conscious control, i.e. it can contradict the athlete's conscious decision to push harder by slowing her down. The nervous system reacts to the data it receives from muscles and 'integrate[s] this information in our actions without even realizing it' (Hutchinson 2018: 111). This means that at the heart of intentionality in aesthetic performance, Barba places a mechanism or a system that can *also* operate on a non-conscious, physiological level – an assertion that supports the earlier observation that intentionality is not always 'entirely intentional'.

'A Cat With Which I have Contact', or Intentionality

Focusing on *sats* entails considering a core element in actional outcomes. This is especially the case with deep somatic and highly technical processes like those found in aesthetic, sport, and skilled labour practices. In such contexts, the lack of or an incomplete *sats* does not only lead to imprecision and errors in execution, but to lifeless (disengaged and mono-tone) movement. This is of critical importance for aesthetic performers like actors and dancers because their bodies are instruments of communication, as distinct from athletes and other skilled individuals whose endeavours are not necessarily tied to corporeal presentation but to results such as a podium finish or a 'personal best'. The distinction that Odin Teatret's Roberta Carreri makes between 'action' and 'movement' gives a sense of the difference that *sats* generates in actional outcomes:

> An action is different from a movement. A movement does not aim physically to change something in the space. An action always wants to produce a change. I shift my notebook: this is an action. I want to change the position of my notebook – that is, I have a precise intention. If it were a suitcase instead of a notebook, then my *in-tension* would be different because my body would have to prepare to lift a heavier weight.
>
> (Carreri 2014: 67, emphasis in the original)

In other words, intentionality is not exclusively a mental phenomenon but is intimately related to muscular activation and its modality.

Although intentionality in such contexts is intrinsically conscious (e.g. one intends to pick *that* object and not something else), muscular activity operates according to differing degrees of automaticity. As elaborated in Part I, an individual may not be fully aware of all the muscles that are engaged

Action, Intention, Transformation   129

when performing specific actions. This is in part due to the recessive nature of muscles and the nervous system but also to the focus requirements of intentionality itself. That is, rather than on which muscles to engage, when, and how, Carreri focuses 'externally' (also in the sense used in Chapter 2) on the notebook to be picked up from the floor. More precisely, she focuses on *picking a book with specific affordances* of weight, size, and texture that automatically through experience determine which muscles are to be activated and to what extent. This tallies with Barba's assessment of the thought-action of *sats* as 'a muscular, nervous and mental commitment, already directed towards an objective' ([1993] 1995: 54).

However, there is more to intentionality than mental and muscular engagement. Referring to Michael Chekhov (1891–1955), a student of Stanislavski who went on to develop the work on the actor's inner life by means of what he called 'psychological gesture', Barba again deploys the word 'innervated'. This time, in addition to the nervous connection between thought and action that characterizes *sats*, he alludes to the sensorial and emotional dimension of the muscular and physiological aspects of actional outcomes: 'everything that he [Michael Chekhov] calls "sensation", "feeling" or "psychological state" is innervated through precise physical attitudes' (Barba [1993] 1995: 76). Therefore, the mental dimension of intentionality is not only integrated with physical engagement but also involves emotional activity. The *body memory* of muscular activation that accompanies the mental mobilization of an intention evokes other phenomena like memories and sensations, all of which carry an emotional charge, however minimal or intense. This picture of action presents a complex and overlapping sequence of events with crucial implications for an understanding of the roles played by sensorial and emotional feelings in psychophysicality. It is worth unpacking some of its layers from the aesthetic performance perspective of Grotowski, whose lifelong work on the sources, characteristics, and qualities of physical action builds on that of Stanislavski before him.

In a 1986 conference in Liège, Grotowski linked the inside/outside quality of impulses when talking about intention:

> In/tension – intention. There is no intention if there is not a proper muscular mobilization. This is also part of the intention. The intention exists even at a muscular level in the body, and is linked to some objective outside you. [...] Intentions are related to physical memories, to associations, to wishes, to contact with the others, but *also* to muscular in/tensions.
>
> (cited in Richards 1995: 96, emphasis in the original)

130 *Performer Training for Actors and Athletes*

Here Grotowski foregrounds the part played by muscular activation and, by implication, the nervous system. In line with his embodied approach, he does not dismiss the somatic dimension of intention in some kind of Cartesian vision of the brute body that does the heavy lifting, dissociated from other processes. Rather, he integrates the mental and muscular aspects of intention and links it – via the consciousness of explicit memories and the less conscious elements of sensorial feelings – with the *associative* capabilities of experience. Hence his evocation of memories always in terms of 'body memory', whether as 'a tool in the actor's process of self-penetration' (i.e. self-discovery) or as 'a tool in the search for one's essence, understood as the most intimate, pre-cultural aspect of the self' (Laster 2012: 211, 213).

In his 1966 Skara Speech, Grotowski elaborates on the kind of connections and implications of associations and memories:

> What is an association in our profession? It is something that springs not only from the mind but also from the body. It is a return towards a precise memory. [...] Memories are always physical reactions. It is our skin which has not forgotten, our eyes which have not forgotten. [...] It is to perform *a concrete act, not a movement* such as caressing in general but, for example, stroking a cat. Not an abstract cat but *a cat which I have seen, with which I have contact.*
>
> (Grotowski [1968] 2002: 225–6, emphasis added)

For Grotowski, therefore, a performer's work on an actional outcome is not limited to its design and functional intentionality but includes the affective dimension, that is, the sensory and emotional relational intensities that energize (breathe life into) the scores and choreographies of performance. For example, *that* book with its specific affordances *because of* or *as if it has* a specific reason, memory, or image. It is the concrete nature or associations of memory, including *the sensations of what they feel like*, that carry the potential emotional charge I am connecting with the mental and physical specificity of intentions. Although Grotowski's practice evolved over the course of his life, in particular its objectives and aesthetic presentation (Wolford 1997: 9–18; Slowiak and Cuesta 2007: 11), the emphasis on the precision of physical actions remained a constant, especially as understood in the broader sense that includes intentions, memories, and emotions.

As such, Grotowski's is an endeavour that recalls Stanislavski's work upon oneself – except, that is, for 'the question of impulses', which Grotowski identified as 'the difference' in their respective investigations on physical action. While Stanislavski concentrated on the restricted remit of social and psychological realism, Grotowski engaged with a wider and more

Action, Intention, Transformation 131

fundamental domain that transcends specific manifestations of life: 'And in such a stream of life the impulses are most important' (Richards 1995: 98–9). The 'question of impulses' brings us back to their importance in Barba's conceptualization of *sats*, in particular in marking the intersectionality of thought, action, sensations, and emotion. To develop the discussion, we now turn our gaze towards the kind of contributions and adjustments made by emotional states to actional outcomes, including their status and timing.

Emotion Modulation

Emotion modulation refers to the regulation or inflection of 'one's emotional response to a situation' (Hogan 2016). As such it overlaps with both the preceding and the subsequent components in an emotion episode, i.e. with the *actional outcome* and its *cognitive processing* respectively. As already noted, the sequence in an episode is not a linear progression of discretely demarcated stages. We are dealing with overlying states or, more precisely, with different aspects and timeframes of the *same phenomenon*, all relating to each other in complex ways. As psychologists Nico H. Frijda and Klaus R. Scherer acknowledge, emotion is 'a multicomponential phenomenon in which the relationships between the component phenomena and the role of each component as a constituent (necessary or sufficient) criterion are far from clear' (in Sander and Scherer 2009: 142).

However contentious it may be, the componentiality or parsing that affective science makes available is grounded in a way that 'intensity', 'incipience', and other terms from affect theory are not, thus rendering amenable for analysis not only emotion and action but also, as seen above, attendant dimensions like intentionality as mental action. On the other hand, affect theory allows the consideration of elements (and *connecting flows*) that are not captured by the filter of affective science. Although lacking visibility, such qualities as 'presence', 'energy', and 'effort' – which elude the categorization of 'affective components' – are nevertheless felt and experienced, especially as magnified (or *intensified*) by practitioners of the body like aesthetic and sports performers.

Emotion modulation is another aspect that lends itself to the cross-lighting of affective science and affect theory. Hogan describes it as the endeavour to 'shift, diminish, sustain, or intensify one's emotional response to a situation *by changing oneself*' (Hogan 2016, emphasis added). I propose foregrounding the point that risks being overlooked in Hogan's syntax, i.e. the *changing of oneself* to modulate one's response. This relation of oneself to oneself is reminiscent of Massumi's understanding of sensations as the

132 *Performer Training for Actors and Athletes*

sensorial feeling of movement in terms of self-referentiality (Massumi 2002: 13–14), which, as discussed in Chapter 4, echoes Matt Fitzgerald's perception of effort as a doubled-layered feeling (emotionally) about how an athlete feels (physiologically) (Fitzgerald 2016: 48; Camilleri 2023).

A literally 'in your face' example of emotion modulation concerns attempts by endurance athletes to regulate their perception of effort – and therefore of *effort itself* – by smiling as a mechanism to contain and counter the negative impact of exertion. This case illustrates the *intersecting characteristics of emotion modulation* for it necessarily operates on the preceding component in an emotion episode, i.e. smiling *during* the ongoing *actional outcome* of running. At the same time, it also overlaps with the subsequent component as it strives to condition the perception, and therefore the *cognitive processing*, of that action.

A recent study by a team of sports and exercise psychologists explored the impact of altering facial expressions (namely, smiling and frowning) and of relaxation (specifically hands and upper body) on 'movement economy, physiological, and perceptual responses during running' (Brick et al. 2018: 20). The study, claiming to be the first of its kind, found that while periodic smiling 'may improve movement economy during vigorous intensity running', mainly through a reduction in heart rate, frowning 'may increase effort perception and [muscular] activation' (2018: 20, 25, 26). The impact of relaxation on 'running economy', i.e. the energy demand and oxygen consumption at a given pace (see Chapter 1), was found to be negligible.

Apart from showing the potential benefits of smiling on one's perception of effort, thus *modulating* one's feeling of and feelings for the ongoing actional outcome, the study's findings on the impact of frowning on muscular activation also informs the discussion on *action readiness*. Despite the negative impact on running economy due to the extra exertion, the 'increased feelings of vigor and energy' that accompanied frowning were deemed to possibly facilitate performance in other contexts such as weightlifting (Brick et al. 2018: 26). In other words, deployed as 'a regulatory strategy in a situationally-appropriate manner' (26), frowning can *prime* the body (i.e. make it *action ready*) for the desired actional outcome.

In both cases, then, the volitional physiological enactment of smiling and frowning triggers a reactive sequence in the body that, in *simulating* the socio-culturally conditioned external manifestation (facial expression) of an internal occurrence like an emotional or muscular event, leads to the actual *stimulation* of that response, in our case, of emotional inflection and/ or corporeal priming. The status of such stimulation can be aligned with Massumi's unacknowledged and unformulated tendencies that reside as

Action, Intention, Transformation 133

residue (as *non-conscious corporeal potential*) when not selected/actualized during the back-formation process of perception (see Chapter 4). Moreover, the relation between external manifestation and internal occurrence of an emotional or muscular state again partakes of the self-referentiality that Massumi ascribes to sensations, which he describes in terms of resonation and echoes (2002: 13–14). Perhaps a more apt image to capture the bidirectionality involved is the reflection of two mirrors in front of each other, where the reflected reality *becomes* the source reality.

Furthermore, as the enactment is *volitional*, that is, knowingly and strategically activated, for example in the context of a competition, on a theatre stage, or even in daily life, this external/internal reiterative mirroring is additionally complicated by the psychological/cognitive layer that *intends* and *wills* it to happen. As evidenced in the distinction between 'I smile *to* feel happy' and 'I smile *because* I feel happy', the end-result of integrated sensorial/emotional feeling of happiness may be similar, but it is the *processual modulation* that differs. I return to the constructed quality of actions and their emotional status in the Conclusion as an important dimension in acting processes but here it suffices to note their capacity to adjust feeling/s.

Changing Oneself

In the bidirectional mirroring of external simulation and internal stimulation, 'the feeling of having a feeling' of sensations overlaps with the *cognitive processing* stage in emotional episodes. Although the cognition of actional outcomes is discussed in Chapter 6, some of its qualities can be anticipated here in the cross-lighting provided by emotion modulation and of examples already evoked in Part II: namely, Kostya's stage fright in Stanislavski and Lindh's mental precision. This discussion complements Neal Utterback's project of enhancing what he calls the 'pre-theatrical' or 'pre-rehearsal' dimension of novice actors via techniques from sports psychology. His pragmatic approach intersects with the simulation–stimulation phenomenon I have identified when he specifically addresses 'power posing' (i.e. 'artificially induced expansive [body] shapes' to boost confidence) and positive 'self-talk' to change one's perception of oneself through self-belief (Utterback 2016: 82). According to Utterback, this hybrid training of 'actor-athletes' is aimed at tackling 'the physical and emotional demands of performing under the pressure of observation' (2016: 92).

In Stanislavski's account, the neophyte actor modulates emotion almost accidentally when he deploys his self-directed rage at the service of the role

134   *Performer Training for Actors and Athletes*

he was playing. Kostya's rage, which he experiences due to the inability to control his body during stage fright, became Othello's:

> I was making a failure, and in my helplessness I was suddenly seized with rage. For several minutes I cut loose from everything about me. I flung out the famous line, "Blood, Iago, blood!" I felt in these words all the injury to the soul of a trusting man. Leo's interpretation of Othello suddenly *rose in my memory and aroused my emotion.*
>
>   (Stanislavski [1936] 1989: 11, emphasis added)

Kostya's friend Leo had moved him emotionally when he had previously spoken about 'the sorrow, the shock, the amazement of the Moor, that such vice could exist in the lovely form of Desdemona' (Stanislavski [1936] 1989: 11). And it was this memory, this *knowledge* that surfaced in his consciousness and stimulated his feelings, which led to Kostya's re-*cognition* and back-formation of a particular 'feeling of having a feeling'. In doing so, he managed to graft that cognitively filtered sensation-of-helplessness-turned-emotion-of-rage onto Othello's. Consequently, in this process of bidirectional mirroring, Kostya *unintentionally* manages to modulate his *own* emotion; that is, a feeling of personal relief at somehow repurposing his rage into Othello's, leading to 'I was full of faith in myself' (12).

If Kostya's fortuitous modulation of emotion features on one side in a spectrum of volition, Lindh's research on mental precision can be located on the other. While resonating with theatre-makers that came before him, especially Grotowski who developed Stanislavski's work on psychophysical action (Richards 1995: 93–9), Lindh's focus on 'mental precision' in a context of collective improvisation sheds a different light on the matter. His insistence on the descriptive term 'mental' rather than 'psychological' is revealing. For him, the term 'psychological' indicates a mechanism (e.g. need, desire, and motivation) that *filters* an action by predetermining it, thus announcing a split where the mind controls the body. The term 'mental' was preferred by Lindh because it excludes psychological mechanisms, in the process highlighting action as an intention to do something without a (psychological) motive to do it (Camilleri 2008b: 430).

In Lindh's research, the action of throwing a stone during an improvisation does not involve the back-forming 'filtering' of a psychological motive to do so, say, like the anger of Kostya's outburst as Othello. Rather, it marks a reaction elicited by *the capacity to listen to a situation.* The legibility of that action (e.g. 'showing anger') occurs *after* its occurrence as an interpretive act. In this sense, Lindh's collective improvisation always aimed at staying one step ahead of a psychology (e.g. motivation) and of procedures (e.g.

Action, Intention, Transformation135

choreography) whose status is predetermining (Camilleri 2008b: 431). The 'capacity to listen to a situation' and act upon it recalls Hogan's account of emotion modulation as a 'response to a situation' (2016). Although in Lindh this response initially marks a physical–mental action, it is subsequently 'read' (i.e. *processed* and *modulated*) also emotionally.

*

The example of emotion modulation foregrounds the intricate relationship between the various components in an emotion episode, including as it involves subsequent stages. As the case of periodic smiling during effortful activity demonstrates, in *intentionally* conditioning actional outcome, these instances involve *cognitive processing* (i.e. the *decision* to smile to alter the outcome) and *phenomenological tone* (i.e. it is *that* tone/feeling itself that sparks the decision to smile/frown *and* which determines whether it was effective or otherwise). To intentionally smile or frown, then, becomes a form of actional outcome in its own right, but it is a scaffolded or intermediary action towards the higher objective of a more effective athletic, aesthetic, or daily performance.

With extensive practice, the processes in the theoretically linear causality of an emotion episode fold in on themselves because what was initially conscious (intentionally worked upon in training to be enacted in performance) becomes automatized to various degrees. In the case of running, the three-way-process of decision–action–effect to smile or frown becomes akin to *and part of* the various integrated aspects of running economy (like balance, stride, cadence, breathing, rhythm, and posture) that cannot be separated from each other.

Notwithstanding the overlapping fusion and bidirectional mirroring of elements in an emotion episode, it remains methodologically worthwhile to consider them individually to spotlight certain operative features that otherwise risk becoming blurred or overlooked. Accordingly, the following chapter attends to cognitive processing and phenomenological tone.

6

Putting on an Act:
Performance Through Experience

Patrick Colm Hogan (2016) acknowledges that 'phenomenological tone', or the subjective feeling of emotions, is the dominant aspect generally associated with emotions. It deals with *what I feel*. As such it is also the most elusive, for I cannot feel *what you feel* because we have different bodies and experiences, different bodyworlds. One way of compensating for this problem is to consider the subjective ineffability of feeling in the light of other components in an emotion episode, in particular of *cognitive processing*. Like Brian Massumi's self-relationality of movement, or 'how I feel feeling' (Massumi 2002: 14; see Chapter 4), cognitive processing marks how we *sense* (perceive) and *make sense of* (understand) feeling.

It is appropriate to consider cognition and feeling together not only because the perception and reading of phenomenal tonality is an embodied form of processing but also because the combination defines the experiential culmination of emotion episodes. As the endpoint in Hogan's categorization of emotion episodes, 'phenomenological tone' marks *what emotionally colours my sensorial feelings*, which is always in the spatio-temporal here and now of occurrence, even if its evolution (as emergent in the other components of an episode) stretch to other times and places. In thus affirming the presence and present-ness of feeling, 'phenomenological tone' is indeed the destination point of emotion episodes.

Accordingly, *cognitive processing* and *phenomenological tone* are considered together in this chapter, with the additional aim of drawing on and integrating various insights from Parts I and II for a more holistic picture. Following an expository discussion on cognitive processing, the chapter proceeds to phenomenological tone via an exemplificatory account from theatre practice that brings together the performing arts and sports, that is, a specific focus on *aesthetic experience in athletic practice*, thus complementing a major undercurrent in the book concerning the *athletic dimension in aesthetic performance*. The title of the chapter reflects this remit, with 'putting on an act' alluding to the aesthetic quality of organized and trained action, and 'performance through experience' referencing the cognitive processing and phenomenological tone of embodiment.

138   *Performer Training for Actors and Athletes*

The basic premise of the chapter is that irrespective of its discipline, genre, and even intention, any performance, whether aesthetic, athletic, or quotidian, is at its most fundamental level 'an act' that involves 'putting on', i.e. requiring preparation and presentation. 'Putting on', which resonates with the sartorial etymology of 'habitational action' discussed in Chapter 4 (cf. Camilleri 2013c), entails training and practice. Although 'putting on an act' may have pejorative connotations of feigning appearance and of exaggerated behaviour, it can be reclaimed in the organizational and aesthetic context of *staging a performance*. Deriving directly from theatre production, the phrase specifically emphasizes the performer's *act*. Consequently, it is associated with the aesthetic performance of actors, dancers, and other performing artists. Beyond the broad territory of performance studies, which views human activity as always already 'putting on an act' or 'acting a part' with reference to gender, ethnicity, class, profession, or other roles humans perform on a daily basis, this chapter extends the emphasis on '*the staging of an act in performance*' to athletic practices.

Cognitive Processing

In the cross-lighting perspective of affect theory and affective science adopted in Part II, *cognitive processing* is where 'affect' as non-conscious relational intensity between body and world develops into the phenomena we recognize and interpret. Such conscious processing, or rather *processing of consciousness*, is selective and therefore *exclusionary* because as much as it endeavours to encompass what is happening (to monitor, evaluate, and predict), it is dependent on the individual's filtering mechanism, on *knowledge* accumulated through experience, whether it is practical '*know how*', reflective '*know* what', or even theoretical/scientific '*know* that' (Nelson 2013: 37).

For a more complex picture of the cognitive activity involved in felt experience, it is worth referring briefly to Part I, which specifically deals with mind–body relationalities in athletic and aesthetic practices. The major aspects covered in Part I include *attentional focus* in Chapter 1, in particular 'internal sensory monitoring' (regarding one's performance), 'self-regulation' of techniques and strategies (vis-à-vis the preparation and planning of performance), and 'outward monitoring' (concerning environmental factors) (Brick et al. 2014: 124). Similar to other explanations in sports science, Noel Brick et al.'s model captures 'distraction' as a form of cognitive processing, whether involuntary or intentional, with the latter signalling a kind of scaffolded organization that conditions how one *feels*

Performance Through Experience 139

about something by *thinking about* something else, thus marking an indirect but intimate connection between thinking and feeling.

Chapter 2 develops the discussion via Gabriele Wulf's (2013) elaboration on internal/proximal and external/distal focus that distinguishes between an athlete's concentration on a moving body part or away from it respectively, thus highlighting other specific modes of cognizing movement. Moreover, the chapter's account of epistemic actions, which describe doing something in an indirect way (such as taking down notes as a memory aid to *do* something or as a critical reflection that informs future *acts*) also resonates with scaffolded-type processing. Chapter 3's consideration of effort perception again involves cognitive filtering, this time in direct relation to 'feeling': from Gunnar Borg's scales that measure RPE (rate of perceived exertion), to Samuele Marcora's 'psychobiological' training aimed at influencing the experience of effort, to John Nietfeld's metacognitive tactics and strategies deployed by athletes to enhance performance.

In Hogan's (2016) account of emotion episodes, cognitive processing can vary from a 'purely informational' acknowledgement of one's body and its immediate environment, to the conditioning of that perception by certain tendencies and states. Applying Hogan's understanding to an outdoors running activity, cognitive processing can involve: (1) *noting* clouds in the sky, including their shape and colour; (2) *assessing* them as either harmless or potentially disruptive in the context of other conditions, for example as they pertain to one's current form, climate, terrain, and the activity in question; and/or (3) *integrating* that information within the dominant sensorial/emotional feeling at the moment. The range of processing marked by *noting*, *assessing*, and *integrating* includes neutral, positive, negative, and emotion congruent cognitions (Hogan 2016).

Consider the case of a runner at the 30 km mark in a marathon (42 km) when it starts to rain from the clouds noticed earlier and as had been forecast. In that closing quarter of the run, when the runner is about to start dipping into her energy and motivation reserves for the final push, her cognitive processing of the event can hardly be as 'purely informational' as it might have been earlier when she registered the material environment. However, even such 'registering' is rarely as 'purely informational' as it is on any given non-running day because already in the first kilometre one is considering (*processing*) ahead the different variables in play, including the possibility of rain, when/where it might occur, as well as measures that can be taken to mitigate for that eventuality, all this while running and noticing (*processing*) other aspects of the situation. When rain hits, the runner can possibly stress, positively, 'generalities over particulars' (Hogan 2016), e.g. that she has already coped optimally with 30 km and 'only' 12 km remain. Or she can

140   *Performer Training for Actors and Athletes*

stress, negatively, 'particulars over generalities' (Hogan 2016), e.g. that her high-stacked footwear will slow her down on the wet roads. Alternatively, she *processes* the rain in her stride (literally), reinforcing her 'predominant emotion at the time' (Hogan 2016), whether she is feeling strong or fatigued.

In this scenario, the runner's *experience* plays a crucial role when processing information. The range and depth of experience allows the athlete to 'back-form', indeed to *re-cognize* (and therefore to process in a specific way), a sensorial/emotional feeling by comparing it to other rainy days and other runs in similar and different conditions. As discussed in Chapter 4, 'back-formation' is Brian Massumi's term for the *always already retrospective* readings involved in cognitive processing. Viewed from this angle of felt perception, cognition enables the supervision and evaluation of the situation as it is unfolding, which in turn colours the overall emotion.

In other words, re-*cognition* provides the basis for re-*experiencing* a sensation and/or emotion. This does not mean experiencing the same feelings all over again (i.e. *processing* feelings the same way) because every situation is materially different *and* because the individual herself evolves dynamically, i.e. she is not the same person she was a week or a year earlier. After all, the fundamental point of experience as an echo chamber of self-relationality (Camilleri 2020a: 27) is the capacity to grow and mature with additional knowledge. Re-*cognition*, therefore, serves as a *reference* for the reading of feeling *through* experience.

In the thick of an endurance event or during the dynamically evolving conditions in sports, when one is completely engaged in the activity, one is not simply *in* but *of* a situation, thus epitomizing 'bodyworld' as explained in the Introduction. Much of the processing in these instances happens rapidly, even at the 'virtual' speeds that Massumi ascribes to body–world relational intensities, that blur the gap between occurrence, perception, decision, and outcome (Massumi 2002: 30), especially in the case of experienced and elite athletes with exceptional degrees of automaticity and flexibility. The 'virtuality' of such processing resonates with enactive approaches to cognition, which assert that activities like perception, understanding, and planning arise from a 'continuous adaptive interplay' between an organism and its environment, including as manifested in athletic practice (Cappuccio 2019: xx).

In the hypothetical case of our marathon runner, the athlete *incorporates* (i.e. she *processes* by *embodying*) the information about the clouds within what sociologist and veteran distance runner John Hockey calls her 'form'. This 'form' *enacts* perception as much as the movement of running:

> When distance runners run they experience 'form' which is the totality
> of their experience as they move over ground. *This totality encompasses*

Performance Through Experience 141

corporeal sensations and linked emotions together with an ongoing cognitive evaluation of those latter two features. This synthesised process combines the *distance running body* with the *distance running mind*, making such experiences fully embodied.

(Hockey 2013: 130–1, emphasis added)

Sensations, emotions, and cognitions all wrapped up in the act of running. Hockey's synthesis of an athlete's body and mind recalls Phillip Zarrilli's psychophysical fusion of an aesthetic performer's bodymind (see Chapter 1). Both Hockey's and Zarrilli's explanations are informed by the enactive approach to cognition (Zarrilli 2020: 12). But that is not the end of the story, for the totality of sensations, emotions, and cognitions 'all wrapped up in running' occurs *in the world*, which is where *bodyworld* comes in.

Hockey's synthesized 'distance running body' and 'distance running mind' does not occur in a vacuum but is inalienably *shaped by* – and indeed *integrated with* – a specific *distance running world* that the individual inhabits, hence the post-psychophysical conceptualization of *bodyworld* and of the *habitational action* it necessitates (Camilleri 2019: xvii). In other words, a runner's 'form' is emergent from the materiality of the event, which includes the world as much as the body.

Enacting Action

On this account, therefore, cognitive processing does not occur independently of the material situation. Neither does it occur independently *within* the individual 'by some dedicated part of the organism that monitors the environment and passes motor instructions on to other parts; rather, it is realized entirely *immanently*, in virtue of the organism's autonomous organization' (Colombetti 2014: 101, emphasis in the original; cf. Murphy 2019a: 84). The nature of that 'immanence', it must be stressed, is in relation to the world. 'Autonomous organization' does not mean 'isolated from the environment, but rather that its interactions with the environment serve to sustain the organism's self-constitution' (Murphy 2019a: 10). This is how theatre practitioner and scholar Maiya Murphy explains the embodied cognitive processing agency of 'actor-creators' who engage with their training and rehearsal environments in ways that resist predetermination (e.g. when working with 'themes, exercises, prompts, instructors, or other actors'; 2019a: 10), thus seeking to *create* rather than merely reproduce meaning. Murphy focuses on Jacques Lecoq's movement practice to illustrate her

142 *Performer Training for Actors and Athletes*

concept of actor-creator, including by tackling some of his principles as discussed in Chapter 4 such as *le jeu* (playfulness), *disponibilité* (openness), and *complicité* (togetherness).

Murphy's choice of a body-based practice like Lecoq's to explore embodied cognitive processes in aesthetic performance is not a coincidence for, unlike 'actor-interpreters [of] psychologically realist text-based work' (2019a: 5), mime work *foregrounds* the sense-making capacities of physicality and movement. There are grounds for a parallel argument to be made that distinguishes technically accomplished '*athlete*-interpreters' from equally proficient '*athlete*-creators' who, because of psychophysiological circumstances, have the ability to change the proverbial name of the game by moving beyond the skills and methods they learnt and mastered. Massimiliano Cappuccio's explanation of sports expertise in terms of a capacity to create 'new' outcomes from reconstituted experiences goes some way in justifying the notion of 'athlete-creators': 'According to enaction theory, expertise is more than just adaptive responsiveness to familiar situations; it also comprises the strategic anticipation of uncertain situations based on the capability to *creatively recombine previous experiences to envision unprecedented forms of resolution*' (Cappuccio 2019: xxxi, emphasis added). This 'creative' dimension is discussed in greater detail later in the context of a specific 'phenomenal tone', but here it suffices to mark connections between enhanced sense-making and specific forms of embodied training. Such training goes beyond the requirement of teaching skills and instead operates holistically on the individual, i.e. not simply learning how to do something mechanically, however well, but also nurturing a capacity to be inventive and flexible in any situation.

Murphy maintains that Lecoq's approach is one such expansive form of training that intervenes on the integrity and autonomy of the individual rather than narrowly on the technique. She adopts the views of affective and cognitive scientist Giovanna Colombetti on 'enactive sense-making and the *simultaneity of cognition and affect*' to explain the 'reciprocity of movement and affect' in Lecoq (Murphy 2019a: 93, emphasis added). In thus highlighting the fundamental union of sensorial and emotional feeling, Murphy identifies it as a foregrounded and key element in Lecoq's approach. Although this is true to various degrees for other psychophysical practices evoked in this book, like those of Decroux, Grotowski, Barba, Lindh, and Zarrilli, Lecoq's emphasis on *state of being* (or frame of mind and 'heart') – as evidenced in *jeu*, *disponibilité*, and *complicité* – provides his practice with a recognizable inflection.

The affective resonance of Lecoq's movement work comes to the fore in what he termed the *mimodynamic* process (Camilleri 2019: 166–7). David

Performance Through Experience 143

Bradby described this aspect of Lecoq's practice as a 'method allowing the actor to discover physical movements which translate into bodily action the sensations aroused in them by colours, words, music' (in Lecoq [1997] 2002: 178). In Lecoq's words:

> Through the mimodynamic process, rhythms, spaces, forces and static objects can all be set in play. Looking at the Eiffel Tower, each of us can *sense a dynamic emotion* and put this emotion into movement. It will be a dynamic combining rootedness with an upward surge, having nothing to do with the temptation to give a picture of the monument (a figurative mime). It's more than a translation: it's an emotion. Etymologically, the word emotion means 'setting in motion.'
>
> (Lecoq [1997] 2002: 48, emphasis added)

In other words, rather than simply teaching movement (e.g. how to walk in terms of balance, alignment, and so on), which he also did, in a mimodynamic modality Lecoq focused on the capacities of observation (and therefore perception) and transformation (or embodied processing) *through* sensorial and emotional experience.

Murphy's reading of enactivism and Lecoq in the light of each other, therefore, foregrounds movement, cognition, and affect as facets of the same phenomenon that reciprocally in/form (i.e. *process*) each other, marking cases where sensorial perception coincides with meaning-making. This brings me to the 'phenomenological tone' of emotion episodes, where sensorial feeling and cognitive processing converge to produce the meaning of *what I feel*. As indicated earlier, reference will be made to 'aesthetic experience' as a channel to evoke the elusive – 'essentially private' and 'ultimately unshareable' (Hogan 2016) – category that is *phenomenological tone*.

Aesthetic Experience

In a recent article, sports lecturer John Toner and former professional ballet dancer now philosophy professor Barbara Gail Montero consider the aesthetic dimension of sports performers. They draw links between an athlete's awareness of certain aspects of her performance (like the design, rhythm, and energy quality of movement) and a dancer's appreciation of the same (2020: 115–16). Toner and Montero also compare this awareness with 'the type of experience one might have in perceiving art: a type of pleasure that is valuable in and of itself' (114). They conclude that not only

144   *Performer Training for Actors and Athletes*

is it justifiable to speak of 'aesthetic judgements' – and therefore of aesthetic interventions – in athletic practice, but that these may matter instrumentally to optimize performance.

The implications of an athlete's *aesthetic* 'awareness' and 'judgement' of her performance include sensory perception, cognitive processing, and actional outcomes. The capacity for 'aesthetic judgement' potentially overlaps with and informs mechanisms and dynamics discussed in previous chapters, whether it is on a physiological level like Tim Noakes's and Ross Tucker's 'anticipatory regulation' that is concerned with maintaining homeostasis (Chapter 3), or on affective science's level of 'emotion modulation' that parallels and conditions actional outcome (Chapter 5).

Although this is not the place to expand on aesthetic reception, the conceptualization of 'aesthetic experience' and its companion 'aesthetic judgement' can be unproblematically situated amongst other regulatory processes. Art often works on subliminal levels, as such it parallels the recessive quality of mechanisms like Noakes's 'anticipatory regulation' that can override explicit conscious control. To shed light on the capacity of 'aesthetic judgement', Tucker's 'template RPE' (2009) can be juxtaposed with Hockey's 'kinaesthetic awareness' or self-image of runners (2013). As expounded in Chapter 3, Tucker's template refers to an athlete's theoretical construct of her Rate of Perceived Exertion during exercise. This subconscious model, which is generated from past experiences and from knowledge about the upcoming task, is continuously compared to the athlete's conscious/actual RPE during the activity. According to Tucker, it enables Noakes's mechanism of 'anticipatory regulation' and explains the contentious claim that it operates beyond conscious control.

In Hockey's case, too, a runner's kinaesthetic self-image is 'forged' in the processes of continuous practice: 'after thousands of training miles one knows sensorially how one is running and one possesses an internal conception of oneself doing so' (2013: 136). This 'sensorial [*know*] how' does not equate the kind of knowledge that smart watches make available, but a 'felt corporeality' that Hockey associates with what philosopher and medical doctor Drew Leder calls the 'visceral body', that is, with 'a visceral understanding based on sensations emanating from moving muscles, ligaments, skin, tendons and organs, particularly lungs' (Hockey 2013: 134).

Therefore, both Tucker and Hockey present modalities of cognitive processing by elite or veteran athletes (i.e. by *experienced* practitioners) that can be described as *embodied*, even *physiological*. Although this processing may not be fully conscious, it does not mean that it is not intentional on a metacognitive level as discussed in Chapter 5, i.e. although a footballer may not be fully conscious of all the muscles she engages when volleying a

Performance Through Experience

ball toward goal, her overall objective and training *is* to score goals; likewise with strategic pacing during a race that depends on the athlete's sense of her situational self (i.e. her bodyworld). The juxtaposition of Tucker's and Hockey's processes suggests the possibility of an *internal template* or *idealized state* consisting of movement shapes and somatic sensations/emotions. Such a template, generated and constantly refined by extensive practice, serves as a measure for what optimal performance should *look* and *feel* like. Consequently, in functioning as a standard or benchmark, this template or idealized image marks an *aesthetic*, precisely of action and feeling.

Such an 'aesthetic' can be aligned with the movement economy of athletes, which varies according to the sports discipline and to individual style. In the section on 'Movement Aesthetic and Economy' in Chapter 1, the *'running economy'* of runners is identified as distinct from the movement economy of other athletes whose discipline may include running (like football and long jump) or not (like swimming and golf). Different sports have different movement economies and, by extension, different aesthetics. The movement economy of a veteran runner, as described in Chapter 1, is made up of form, specifically all her *experiences of form*, which include not only her background, training, and races, but other aspects of knowledge like those she may have read about and observed in other athletes. It is precisely this knowledge or 'standard' that becomes an *aesthetic*, and when that standard is embodied, the *experience* can be said to be 'aesthetic', including when adapting, adjusting, and altering one's style and technique similar to what inventive and creative *artists* do in their respective fields.

Such experiences are aesthetic in a similar way that Zarrilli ascribed to psychophysical practitioners when writing about the 'aesthetic inner bodymind' they cultivate through deep practice (see Chapter 1). This 'aesthetic inner bodymind', which should not be confused with what Zarrilli calls the 'aesthetic outer body' (i.e. the persona that spectators see on stage), functions on a level that resonates with an internalized template or idealized sensorial image that athletes develop over time. An actor's or a dancer's 'aesthetic inner bodymind', therefore, is a felt awareness and experience of her body that is not necessarily fully conscious, and that shapes the 'aesthetic outer body'. As such, an aesthetic performer's bodymind and an athlete's sensitized template – both of which mark inner modulating capacities that evolve with practice – can be considered as different inflections of the same *phenomenological tone* that are here being denoted by 'aesthetic'. To convey a more particular sense of this aesthetic phenomenological tonality, the following sections adopt a different – more subjective and allusive – approach, that involves a number of case studies with improvisation as a key component of experience.

Experience Case Studies

Since 'experience' is a crucial aspect of the current discussion, it is apt to engage – and *enact* – a methodological shift that illustrates the embodied relation between cognition and feeling in somatic practice. Accordingly, I will refer to my experience as a theatre practitioner and runner via a number of case studies.

Without placing myself as arbiter, but also without ignoring my over three decades of theatre practice and twenty-plus years of running (see Preface), my experience suggests very close affinities between the 'phenomenological tone' of certain fundamental instances in theatre and in running, to the extent that both *feel* the same except for modalities related to the different disciplines. Although this equivalence may well be attributable to the quality of optimal performance in both camps and to the ipseity (the selfhood or sense of oneself) of the same experiencer, I have not felt this tonality in other spheres of life. As such, the active variables associated with this shared phenomenological tonality pertain to *the mastery of skills in deep psychophysical practices*.

The following case study reflections about my practice, which are aimed at shedding light on features of phenomenological tone that are more universally applicable, can be located at the methodological intersection of three main movements:

(1) *practice (as) research* in the performing, visual, and other creative arts (Barrett and Bolt 2009; Smith and Dean 2010), where the praxis of the 'practitioner-researcher' is the main instigator and medium of the investigation (Nelson 2013: 25–34);
(2) *'thick description' accounts* from anthropology's observation of human behaviour and its context (Geertz 1973), including as applied to aesthetic performance (Allain 2016); and
(3) *autoethnographic approaches* where 'the researcher's phenomenological experience of engaging with the activity under study' illuminates wider sub-/cultural aspects (Allen Collinson 2005: 224; cf. Duncan 2004: 29–31), including with reference to distance running (Hockey 2013: 128–30).

Zarrilli's writings about performer processes, which combine phenomenological, enactive, and praxis perspectives as the main methodologies, illustrate an example of such intersectional organization, including as presented in his extensive 'Production Case Studies' in *Psychophysical Acting* (2009: 113–211) and 'First-person Accounts of Embodied Practice' in *(Toward) A Phenomenology of Acting* (2019: 20–72).

Performance Through Experience 147

Case Study 1 (Training): Plastiques

Although elusive to express in words, the specific 'aesthetic' feeling or tone in question that still occasionally features in my theatre work and running is neither general nor vague but has a distinct phenomenological quality I have come to recognize. It tends to occur in instances of release or 'letting go', typically in improvisation sessions with techniques or structures that have been mastered after a practice of assimilation and maturation, where I feel at once *liberated by* and *from* that training. This tonality, which, as explained in Case Study 2, I eventually called 'dynamic aliveness', was initially a nameless sensation when it first emerged.

I experienced this phenomenon for the first time early on in my development as an actor, around six years after I started training in 1989, which meant that I already had a solid base of praxis inspired by yoga, acrobatics, and martial arts, as well as by devising and performing in at least four group performances. It was during my quasi-obsessive rendering of Grotowski's plastique exercises, which are based on the organic fragmentation of the body (Slowiak and Cuesta 2007: 137–40), that something techno-phenomenological mobilized in my relation to embodied action.

At this point in my first decade of training, when I was still on a steep learning curve as a performer, I was spending hours on fragmenting the body in terms of left/right, up/down, forward/backward, and anti-/clockwise quarter, semi-circular, circular, and figure-of-eight movements of different body parts whilst trying not to move the rest. The major elements in this fragmentation included the head, neck, shoulders, elbows, wrists, knuckles, fingers, sternum, various points along the spine, knees, heels, and feet. The next step was to connect the fragmented segments to each other, e.g. a micro impulse from the coccyx that travelled up the spine towards the right shoulder that went through the right arm via elbow, wrist, and hand to the tip of the fingers, and back again the same way to the initiating shoulder, circling around the neck to then go either to the other arm via the same itinerary or down the spine to the legs, etc. It was a work of quasi-obsessive precision regarding what I deemed as the 'grammar' of a particular exercise. Aspects of this technique can be seen in some of the short training films in *Physical Actor Training: An Online A–Z*, including those I lead on 'Articulation' and 'Hands' (Allain et al. 2018).

I compare the technical device of up, down, left, right, forward, backward, and circular movements at different speeds and in various rhythms to the 'abstraction' of the alphabet in language or the scales in music, hence the reference to the 'grammar' of performance behaviour that can then be layered with other qualities. In fact, the next step of the exercise involved *improvising* with this fragmentation technique, initially by 'playing' with the sequence

148   *Performer Training for Actors and Athletes*

of the connections between parts as my body pulsated with movement, including having more than one initiating impulse generating movement across the body. Later improvisations sought to adopt recognizable gestural shapes by incorporating the plastique impulses into actions such as picking up an imaginary flower, throwing an imaginary stone, kicking an imaginary ball, or smoking an imaginary cigarette. These were all actions that could possibly feature in a performance, which means that, aesthetically, I was working *towards* rather than *from* realist behaviour, in the process prioritizing inner feeling and enaction rather than outward-directed imitation.

Improvising in this way also meant exercising – and therefore *processing through embodiment* – other elements that are not exclusively physical, such as imagination and intention. This meant that on top of the basic image and intention of moving, rotating, and connecting parts of the body, I was now layering more sophisticated levels of cognitive organization when engaging with *imaginary* flowers, stones, balls, and cigarettes. This complexity was further developed with the composition of '*little narrative sequences*' or '*little dramaturgies*' of actions, e.g. picking up a pebble from the floor, feel it around my hand, then throw it like a dart toward a wall, react as if I was hit by the pebble I had just thrown, circle it around inside my torso undulating the spine, then push it out through the arm (articulating shoulder, elbow, wrist, hand, and fingers along the way) like a rabbit out of a magician's hat, etc. 'Like a dart' or 'like a rabbit out of a hat' are the kind of images that shaped the thought-action and intentionality of my behaviour, *modulating* it accordingly as discussed in Chapter 5.

The technique I had assimilated during the 'abstract' stage of the exercise (its 'alphabet' or 'scales') thus also (in)formed the *precision of imagination and intentionality*. Indeed, this technical and improvisation training facilitated the *meaningful* inhabitation of physical and vocal scores – *how I performed* them – by *living* and not merely 'mechanically reproducing' the material. In this regard, and as discussed in the Introduction, I was working on what Franco Ruffini calls the reality and truth of *azione in vita* (action in life) (Ruffini 1995: 54). Performance structures of this sort – irrespective of their aesthetic during improvisation training – come with the sophisticated organization and dynamics of, amongst others, motifs, themes, plot lines, characterizations or role development, and interaction, all of which recall the 'metacognitive' strategies referred to earlier in the context of competitive athletics.

Moreover, my practice of starting from and layering impulses (inspired by Grotowski and Barba) foregrounded sensorial feeling as a material *and* imaginative activity, i.e. as actual *and* 'as if' actions. In other words, the perception of the immediate surroundings of the training studio (e.g. smelling

Performance Through Experience 149

or touching the wooden floor) and imaginatively transforming it in my consciousness into something else (e.g. a forest floor or a prison cell) was an integral part of the plastiques improvisations. Equally significant, along with the enactment of actions, this training *with* and *of* the senses served as a way of accessing and stimulating *memory*, e.g. the studio's wooden floor as imaginatively transformed into a playground could recall a specific place from childhood where a particular event was experienced. The evocation of memories through *sensorial feeling* thus prepared the ground for *emotional feeling* to *emerge* and *modulate* the work, again enabling me to *live* rather than mechanically reproduce the actions I was performing.

Therefore, the nuance of imagination and the decisiveness of intentionality (both of which constituted an integrated phenomenon prompted by the fluent movement of the plastiques) led to a simultaneous mobilization of memories and their related feelings, precisely through what in Chapter 5 is discussed in the context of Grotowski's work on 'the associative capabilities of experience' and 'body memory'. One aspect of such 'associations' was the *lack of predetermination* in both the individual images and the 'little dramaturgies' which layered the fragmentation of the body. On the contrary, these were allowed to emerge and flow as organically as the movement. Whenever the imagination (of a made-up image or an actual memory) dried up, I fell back on the intentionality of the 'abstract grammar' of the exercise until others arose. With time, this practice generated its own memories, i.e. it cultivated the resonance (the *experience*) of working with memories, not only with reference to the individual images themselves (e.g. of *that* specific playground memory from childhood) but, more importantly, to the enhanced *capacity* and *ability* to evoke them. In other words, not simply 'learning something', but *learning to learn*.

Two things need bearing in mind in the context of the work that has been thickly described here. First, the development of the plastiques from one stage to the next was not as linear and logical as it might come across in writing. It was messier and more pragmatic in reality, a 'seeing it feelingly in the dark'. Second, the plastiques were not my only training at the time. Albeit a major element, they formed an integral part of other theatre exercises and devising work (on my own, within a group, and in workshops with other practitioners), including extensive readings and observations of live and filmed training and performances. Moreover, I pursued other physical practices to support my theatre work, including periodic interests such as martial arts and dance to address certain aspects of my development (e.g. balance, footwork, rhythm), as well as ongoing activity for overall muscular flexibility and toning like yoga, light weights, and, very relevant to my argument here, running, specifically short 6 km/30-minute runs about two

150   *Performer Training for Actors and Athletes*

or three times weekly. This bigger picture of my activity sheds further light on the nature of the technical and aesthetic experiences that were also feeding into the plastiques-based improvisation. For example, a plastiques-generated actional outcome from the image of 'kicking an imaginary ball' would be (in)formed, consciously or otherwise, not only by my childhood experience of playing football but also via the embodied memories of martial arts kicks and of running.

Case Study 2 (Training Performance): *Tekhnē Sessions*

The space between mastered technique and playful improvisation, therefore, provided the conditions of possibility for a specific phenomenological tone to emerge in my theatre training, aspects of which I recognize in certain instances when running. Crucially, this is also the cognitive processing space of 'mental precision' as explored by Ingemar Lindh (see Chapter 5). Although I did not work with Lindh on plastiques, he was one of my teachers at the time, right up until his death in 1997 during a workshop I was attending (Camilleri 2008b: 426). Lindh's views on improvisation as performance (Lindh 2010; Camilleri 2008a) were as influential to my formation as Grotowski's on the psychophysical state and Barba's on physical and vocal training.

Apart from my interpretation of the plastiques, the other landmark instance where I perceived this phenomenological tonality was whilst working on the training/performance structure of *Tekhnē Sessions* in the early 2000s. With more experience under my belt as performer and teacher, and leading my theatre group Icarus Performance Project (Malta), I had embarked on a research project investigating the space between training and performance processes. With hindsight, this research can be viewed as a systematic attempt to learn more about the plastiques phenomenon described above because its vitality felt essential to 'being performer'.

Consequently, *Tekhnē Sessions* was intentionally developed as a 'performance structure of training', i.e. *a training* that was presented as *a performance*. Around twenty presentations were given in over three months to small audiences (maximum 20) with the aim of stimulating the appropriate conditions that hybridized the regularity and intimacy of 'training' with the occasionality and exposure of 'public performance'. Co-created with my trainees and co-founders of Icarus, *Tekhnē Sessions* (Camilleri 2004: 4) consisted of three movements that progressively explored different modes of improvisation: from the highly codified dynamic yoga-like and martial-arts-like form of the first movement, to the flexible structure of the second movement (e.g. the task of finding as many body positions as possible while holding the palms of the hands flat on the floor), to the free improvisation of the third movement. It was this final section of *Tekhnē Sessions*, named 'Flight', that frequently generated a feeling or experiential state reminiscent of the plastiques (Figure 1).

Briefly, 'Flight' involved:

> the recall of actions, dynamics, positions, rhythms and other elements from the first two movements. This improvisational recall [took] the form of a selection and adaptation of elements from the practitioners' assimilated techniques, including exercises not incorporated in *Tekhnē Sessions*. The practitioners' concern here [was] not '*what* to do' or '*how* to do' (both of which [were] embodied as residue from the first and second movements) but 'to do compositionally'.
>
> (Camilleri 2018b: 309, emphasis in the original)

Similar to the case of the plastiques, therefore, the conditions of possibility for the phenomenological tonality in question to emerge revolved around technique within a structure, specifically the transcendence-through-mastery of *both* the individual's technique *and* the organizing structure

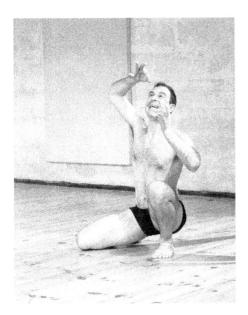

Figure 1 Third Movement of *Tekhnē Sessions* by Icarus Performance Project (ActionBase Studio, Malta, 2004). Photo by Sandro Spina.

152 *Performer Training for Actors and Athletes*

that framed it. Achieved through long-term practice, this is a technical and structural mastery not only in terms of *physical* precision but as integrated within an engagement of mental and affective capacities, i.e. as they pertain to the *attentional, imaginative,* and *emotional* dimensions.

The techno-phenomenological quality I experienced in the 'Flight' section of *Tekhnē Sessions* is something that, five years later, I tried to capture by the term 'dynamic aliveness' (Camilleri 2010: 158–60). In that article, I cross-referenced 'dynamic aliveness' with Zarrilli's psychophysical bodymind (2009), Philip Auslander's micro-relationships of presence (cited in Shepherd and Wallis 2004: 234), and Barba's pre-expressive physical/muscular micro-techniques (see Chapter 1). More recently (Camilleri 2018b: 308–9), I pondered 'dynamic aliveness' in the light of a magnetism of presence via Joseph Roach's materiality of '*it*', referring to the performer's accessories, clothes, and body (2007: 8), and Jane Goodall's 'vibrant aliveness', where the inner and outer dimensions of the actor resonate (2008: 39). However, the etymological implications that originally inspired the name '*tekhnē*' (skill, craft, or method of doing), especially as related to *poiesis* (a produced object), *physis* (nature of being), and *alētheia* (truth as un-concealment), still come closest to evoke this elusive but very real feeling during practice (Camilleri 2018b: 310).

Case Study 3 (Running): Long Runs

Something akin to the phenomenology of 'dynamic aliveness' occasionally features in my running, specifically with regard to movement economy. Running economy consists of aspects such as cadence (steps per minute), stride (length of step), foot strike (the part of the foot that hits the ground first), muscular activation, breathing qualities, rhythm, positioning of the spine, balance (including reduced vertical and horizontal oscillation), and overall generation and flow of energy (see Chapter 1). If *improvisation* brought all techno-phenomenological elements together in my plastiques and 'Flight' manifestations of 'dynamic aliveness', the closest equivalent in running is *pacing* as described in Chapter 3. However, this is a specific expression of pacing, one that is not captured by data that a smart watch makes available because it relies entirely on *feeling*.

Confronted by the challenge of explaining what Hogan called the 'ultimately unshareable' nature of phenomenological tone, a possible alternative to convey a sense of 'dynamic aliveness' in running is not through an account of *what it is* but, rather, by a *via negativa* approach of *what it is not* (cf. Grotowski [1968] 2002: 17, 19). To begin with, it is *not* another term for

Performance Through Experience   153

the so-called 'runner's high', which denotes an elusive sense of euphoria that is sometimes experienced during or *after* a long run (Dietrich and McDaniel 2004: 536). Despite some inevitable overlaps pertaining to long-distance running, the phenomenology of a 'runner's high' (as studied, for example, by Whitehead 2016: 183–5) does not fully match the 'technical awareness' of my experience. Although partaking of them, the running equivalent of 'dynamic aliveness' is also *not* solely about the technique, effort, intention, and awareness of movement economy. For example, the centrality of effort perception is temporarily underwhelmed (rather than 'overwhelmed') by a *quietness of feeling* during 'dynamic aliveness' while running. Just as 'dynamic aliveness' in my plastiques improvisations is characterized by 'going beyond technique', in running this 'quietness of feeling' functions as a kind of 'focus that transcends focus'.

The quietness of this feeling or focus can be partly aligned with Hockey's running modality of the 'almost quiet', that is, a lack of 'chatter' when 'the running body interact[s] with the running mind', when consciousness does not flag up any problems (2013: 133–4). This is not a subdued but an affirmative and affirming silence because, crucially, the runner is in excellent form. Consequently, it only superficially and partly overlaps with the rarefied experience described in Chapter 1 of Haruki Murakami's 'very still, quiet feeling' during his 100 km ultramarathon (2008: 114). The key difference between Murakami's and my experience is *form*: while in Murakami the 'quietness' arose from a *deterioration* of form due to extreme fatigue, in my case it accompanies a *generative fulfilment* of form. Despite this fundamental difference, however, both phenomena share a 'passing clean through' (Murakami 2008: 112) or 'going beyond' – indeed a *disarming of* – a state of consciousness.

Similar to my theatre practice, I have experienced this running state mostly in training, specifically during solo long runs of over 30 km, very early in the morning (circa 3 a.m.), on familiar but deserted roads, particularly in the first 90 minutes or so. These constitutive variables of the experience are revealing, especially the last one because it indicates not only 'physiological actuality' but also 'physiological expectation' as a condition of possibility before intense effort starts building up. 'Physiological expectation' may be related to the subconscious mechanism of 'anticipatory regulation' that enables athletes to maintain biological stability while adjusting to external conditions. A regular 90-minute run does not generally generate the same *feeling* of the first 90 minutes in a much longer run, which indicates a 'quietness' of acceptance while still in peak form. This is different from Murakami's deconstructive 'quietness' that impacted his running economy beyond the 75 km mark of his ultramarathon. Moreover, his running aesthetic was also affected by the ungainly swinging of arms as a momentum-propellant for his aching legs (Murakami 2008: 114). A crucial dynamic to consider here, of course, is pacing, which determines the difference in perception, effort, and output between long and much longer runs (see Chapter 3).

The early morning timing is equally significant, not only because there is less to *occupy* the mind in familiar and traffic-free roads, but because the body memory of sleep at that hour is an effective pacifier of internal chatter, functioning as an 'inverted distraction' in *distracting me from distraction*, hence another form of *embodied processing*. As discussed in Chapter 1, voluntary and involuntary modes of distraction are an integral part of an athlete's attentional focus in endurance exercise, sometimes deployed strategically to enhance performance by diverting the focus away from the pain of exertion, and sometimes activated spontaneously as part of the monitoring processes that note ambient conditions like pleasant scenery. Whenever I experience 'dynamic aliveness' during early morning long runs, the boundary between focus and distraction feels blurred. Such 'inverted distraction', which is another facet of the 'focus that transcends focus', results in this *via negativa* kind of consciousness, i.e. an awareness by elimination of *what it is not*.

Regarding the early morning variable, my own demonstration of work at the Workcenter of Jerzy Grotowski and Thomas Richards, at their base in Pontedera (Italy) in 1996, was held at midnight during a sharing of training and performance material between them and our theatre group (led by our director John J. Schranz). Apart from the uniqueness of the occasion, especially since Grotowski himself was in attendance, presenting at that hour and in those circumstances felt like inhabiting a liminal space–time between wakefulness and sleep, where the self's ever-vigilant physiological and socio-cultural defences are lowered enough to enable a 'clean through' and uncluttered consciousness.

It is important to bear in mind that, even if all the variables mentioned above are present, not every first 90 minutes of an early morning long run result in 'dynamic aliveness'. The *variability* of the connections between these elements, *and* the presence of a multitude of others that range from meteorological conditions to nutritional and emotion states, play a part in processing the felt tonality of a runner's phenomenological bodyworld. What these variables indicate, rather, are a few features that recur in certain instances of 'dynamic aliveness'. Running very early in the morning, then, in the particular conditions of the material environment *and* in optimal form, my consciousness is – *feels* – pacified as I 'pass clean through' the streets. No wonder that in my running log I describe the initial section of such long runs as 'meditational'.

Performance Through Experience 155

Case Study Reflections: Aesthetics in Athletics

In the Introduction I propose the neologism of 'aesthletic' (combining 'aesthetic' and 'athletic') to capture those socio-cultural qualities generally associated with notions of grace, beauty, symmetry, or even form that trained *bodies* possess or acquire in the course of their practice. But what about the relevance of the same notions to the *movement* in athletic endeavour?

As noted in Chapter 1, even if athletic behaviour is not generally driven by aesthetic considerations, the most efficacious expressions of movement economy are likely to be perceived not only in terms of performance output but also according to criteria of style and finesse, such as the balance, design, posture, movement flow, and patterns of play. Although the absolute priority for athletes and fans remains to win, ideally this should be done convincingly rather than 'ugly' (Toner and Montero 2020: 119). Admittedly a secondary consideration, this nevertheless important factor constitutes *aesthetic judgement*. The present chapter contemplates such experiences as 'aesthetic' from the performer's perspective to exemplify a specific case of phenomenological tone that I have identified as 'dynamic aliveness'. As Toner and Montero argue, 'aesthetically pleasing form might matter instrumentally [because] it might contribute to optimal performance' (2020: 113) and my experience of 'dynamic aliveness' during long-distance running appears to back this up. To support this claim, the running equivalent of 'dynamic aliveness' can be aligned with Hockey's understanding of an athlete's experience of form, which he associates with a term that British runners sometimes refer to as the 'going', e.g. 'I'm going well' or 'I'm going badly'.

Hockey's 'going' refers to a sensuous rather than a cognitive kind of 'self-knowledge [that] allows runners to evaluate their athletic endeavours' (2013: 131). Drawing on John Dewey's understanding of aesthetics as an *intensification* of ordinary experience ([1934] 1980), which entails constant adaptation to the situating environment, Hockey considers a runner's judgement of her form as *aesthetic*: 'the sensory-based perceptions of immersion in training are [...] used by runners to categorise their movement: in that sense, they are making aesthetic judgements' (2013: 130).

For Hockey, a runner's judgements such as 'going well' or 'going badly' are the consequence of cognitive processing that mobilizes the major elements discussed so far, i.e. the effort that runners make is '*felt, then perceived and subsequently evaluated* cognitively to arrive at an aesthetic judgement of "going"' (2013: 131, emphasis added). The processual progress from *effort* to *perception* to *cognition* to *judgement* should be viewed in the light of the extended argument developed over the last three chapters, involving the complex overlapping and bidirectional relationality between unconscious

156   *Performer Training for Actors and Athletes*

body-and-world intensities/affects, their sensory perception through enaction, and the eventual emergent emotions that are back-formed by experience.

Hockey's autoethnographic account categorizes (*judges*) the felt perception of his training in three principal ways – 'brill(iant)', 'ok', and 'crap' (2013: 137). He assesses these experiences in terms of 'a series of inter-linked binary oppositions', each consisting of a 'spectrum of embodied knowledge', including soft/hard and heavy/light muscular sensations, the noisy/quiet chatter between body and mind already mentioned, flowing/faltering rhythm, and compact/disjointed postural positioning (131–5). For all intents and purposes, these are aesthetic criteria that apply to athletic performance.

Toner and Montero develop Hockey's experiential spectrums into meta-categories that can apply to a wider range of sports, mainly: (1) 'flying along' (Hockey's phrase for 'flow') to capture a quality of energy; (2) power, as it relates to the muscular force (mainly but not exclusively as generated by the legs); (3) rhythm, as pertaining to movement, breath, and the interplay between different body parts; and (4) the all-encompassing 'feeling right' (Toner and Montero 2020: 118–23). The latter's elusive (and allusive) nature epitomizes Hogan's description of phenomenological tone as well as resonates with my understanding of 'dynamic aliveness':

> "feeling right" represents a general aesthetic evaluation that is commonly used by highly-skilled performers during both practice and competitive performance. It feels right [...] because it hits the aesthetic sweet spot. What exactly this is might not be easy to quantify because the years of training have enabled skilled athletes to chunk vast amounts of information about their skills into higher level concepts; "smooth," or "streamlined," or "like a torpedo" are aesthetic concepts that might capture a decade of information about how to perform a skill.
>
> (Toner and Montero 2020: 122)

It is thus also in this synthesized sense that what stimulates and shapes phenomenological tone also affects its clarity and hinders its share-ability to others. 'Feeling right' is an aspect of what Toner and Montero qualify as the 'positive aesthetic experience' in athletic performance that I am associating with the subjective feeling of 'dynamic aliveness'. They distinguish such phenomenological tonalities from 'negative aesthetic experiences', which are also of instrumental value to an athlete's performance, e.g. the feeling of muscle exhaustion and pain as reference points for endurance athletes (Toner and Montero 2020: 113).

Performance Through Experience   157

The discussion on the phenomenology of my running practice focused exclusively on training as distinct from racing. This is due to the fact that I have not felt this particular quality in competitive conditions. Although the reason for this may reflect my limited experience in running races, mainly because I subscribe to Vybarr Cregan-Reid's view of running as an autotelic activity (2016: 146), I have more than enough embodied knowledge of the kind of elements that frame competitive racing. That is, the active presence of an additional set of complex and evolving variables that potentially restrict (and at times stimulate in equal measure) the conditions of possibility that are operative in training practice. To provide some indication of the phenomenological tone under review in a public performance setting – and therefore shedding some 'side-light' on that aspect of race-running – I refer to theatre performance in the concluding case study.

Case Study 4 (Performance): *Id-Descartes* and *Martyr Red*

Although 'dynamic aliveness' in my theatre practice featured mostly in training situations (including in the hybrid presentations of *Tekhnē Sessions*), I have experienced a related phenomenon in public performances. The two main instances that stand out in this regard are the 'dream sequence' in *Id-Descartes* (1996–2003) and the 'flagellation' scene in *Martyr Red* (2013), both belonging to a style that falls under the broad umbrellas of 'devised' and 'physical' theatre (Murray and Keefe 2016). Various elements that have already been identified in training circumstances recur in these two episodes, including the technical proficiency and assimilation of structures that come with repeated practice, as well as the solo dynamic that frames the events and which allows for a degree of improvisation. *Id-Descartes* was a solo performance, co-created with John J. Schranz as director, and while *Martyr Red* was a co-devised duo with Judita Vivas, the scene in question consisted of a juxtaposition of two independent scores (Icarus Performance Project 2022).

Rather than reconfirm the overlaps with training, it is more effective to home in on additional insights that such performance instances contribute to 'dynamic aliveness': namely that, with experience, I was able to *stimulate* or *trigger* the phenomenological state in question at the relevant point in the respective scores. That is, unlike the improvisation-based structures of the plastiques and *Tekhnē Sessions*, where the tonality emerged quasi-serendipitously (e.g. during a particular body position or a movement rhythm that sparked the feeling), a performance score is more tightly configured. After noting its re-occurrence at the same point in the performance, I discovered that I could initiate and sustain a phenomenological state that recalls 'dynamic aliveness'. Such triggers could be anything from a kind of un/focused look that sparked an equivalent state (i.e. a form of concentration not directed towards anything specific while still being highly aware of what is happening), or a certain tonality or inflection of the voice while singing the phonetic combination of vowels and consonants (and therefore *not* the meaning) of a phrase in a specific rhythm that required a particular body engagement.

My task, which became incorporated in the internal logic and structures of the scores, was to ensure that I was psychophysically and technically prepared – also in a way that recalls 'action readiness' from Chapter 4 – for the moment during the performance to activate the trigger. The task-based organization of the dream sequence and the flagellation scene also helped: this meant that they possessed some freedom, permitting a degree of improvisation as long as the action was fulfilled according to a few space/time criteria that connected with the preceding and subsequent sections of the scores. For example, the dream sequence in *Id-Descartes* was based on a song that I had to sing while moving from lying down on my back to standing up (Figure 2). How and at what speed I transitioned between the levels was

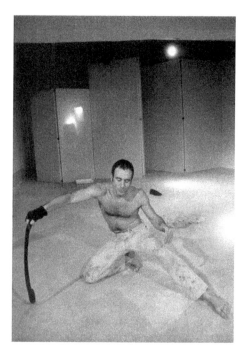

Figure 2 *Id-Descartes* by Groups for Human Encounter (ActionBase Studio, Malta, 2001). Photo by Jeremy de Maria.

up to me as long as I abided by the durational and rhythmic constraints of the song. More relevantly to the 'trigger' mechanism was the care (*attentional focus*) I had to engage to mobilize my body in ways that retained a constant circulation of breath for the song. With practice I discovered that by using vocal impulses at certain points of the song (i.e. using specific syllables as 'pegs') I could shift smoothly from one physical level to another (e.g. from lying down to sitting on the floor to kneeling on one leg) without interrupting the flow of the action. It is precisely the feeling during this seamless *transitional* engagement that reminds me of 'dynamic aliveness'.

In the 'flagellation' scene of *Martyr Red*, after smearing with red lipstick three diagonal lines across the full length of my bare torso and another on top of them (Figure 3), I had to flog my back with an imaginary whip. During the act of self-flagellation, I had to keep the lower part of my body (waist down) locked and immobilized in a wide horse-riding stance (Figure 4), while my torso pivoted around sharply ('violently') as I lashed the whip and felt it land on my back from the flanks or from above my shoulders in various single or double blow combinations (Figure 5). The flogging action was enacted by my stretched arms serving as 'whips' in movements that recalled *plastiques fragmentation* as the swivelling tension between the unmoving legs and moving torso generated the impulse in the centre (in the region just below the navel) that spread to shoulders, elbows, wrists, and gripping hands.

The main constraints of the flagellation scene involved staying in the same centre stage left spot (while my colleague was performing her solo

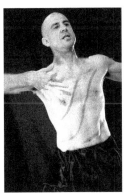
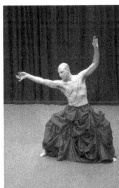
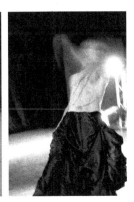

Figures 3, 4, 5 *Martyr Red* by Icarus Performance Project. Figures 3 and 5: Valletta Campus Theatre, Malta, 2013, photo by Jeremy de Maria. Figure 4: Jarman Building, University of Kent, UK, 2013, photo by Icarus Performance Project.

sequence centre stage right) for the circa 2-minute duration of techno music superimposed by a reading of T. S. Eliot's sadomasochistic fantasy 'The Love Song of St Sebastian'. These parameters allowed for a degree of improvisation, including the sequencing of the lashings and their speed, usually starting with a lash every three or so seconds to climax to as many as I could muster per second, before stopping abruptly at the end of the music clip. Like running, I had to *pace* myself not to reach exhaustion level too early. However, it was the progressive acceleration of pivoting around the centre that sparked what I am aligning with 'dynamic aliveness', exactly when bracing myself to start picking up pace, and therefore concentrating on retaining my stance by not moving the legs while the torso swivelled rapidly with the 'whipping' arms flying around, risking to throw me off balance.

While writing this account, and therefore further cognitively processing an aspect of my aesthetic practice, I experienced a case of Nelson's *know what* knowledge that reflects on practical *know how*. The reference to the 'plastiques fragmentation' in the context of the flogging arm movement in *Martyr Red* is significant. That particular engagement of the arms – in terms of psychophysical and technical modality – must have tapped into my body memory of the arm plastiques to stimulate or re-awake the sense of 'dynamic feeling' that frequently accompanied the movement when working on that exercise. This is a feeling and an awareness that I can re-*cognize*.

And yet, the feeling of 'dynamic aliveness' in a performance structure does *not* have the same tonality that occurs in a training improvisation because the outcomes are *not* identical. Compared to the more sustained manifestation in training, the prescribed and often limited duration of the state in performance is indicative of this difference. As I observed in my most recent articulation on the subject: 'My understanding of "dynamic aliveness" *is* related to the materiality of physicality and its accessories […], but rather than referring to a display-oriented showing or performance event I specifically locate it within a training context and associate it with a *composition-in-the-moment* quality' (2018b: 309, emphasis in the original). In the context of the plastiques and *Tekhnē Sessions*, I associate this feeling with the *generation of material*, whether it is an action or a sequence of actions or even a dynamic, rhythm, or pattern that has the 'sense' (sensorial and semantic) of something newly created or configured, hence *composition-in-the-moment*. The structure of a performance score restricts the embodied sense-making frame of composition-in-the-moment that characterizes improvisation in training. This difference in bodyworld conditions is reminiscent of the one between a 90-minute run and the first 90 minutes of a much longer run: although the duration may be the same, the more open process of the longer run or of a

Performance Through Experience   161

training improvisation is key to the exploratory play without the pressure of the imperative to retain the audience's attention. Accordingly, I conclude the chapter with an examination of the *compositional dimension* I am linking with 'dynamic aliveness'.

Improvisational Conclusions

It is possible to contemplate the techno-phenomenological tone of 'dynamic aliveness' in the light of Mihaly Csikszentmihalyi's optimal 'flow' experience as discussed in Chapter 2. There are various correspondences between the two phenomena, including the fusion of action and awareness, total immersion in the doing, and the autotelic status of the activity (Jackson 1996: 76–7). Rather than work through the parallels, I will cut to the chase and focus on the *compositional* factor as the main distinguishing feature between 'dynamic aliveness' and flow.

Although the optimal performance of flow is a creative and generative force, it does not *necessarily* and *always* result in compositional material or organization. Moreover, the compositional dimension I associate with the plastiques and *Tekhnē Sessions* implies an agility or *dynamism* of consciousness and behaviour that is not foregrounded enough in the quasi-passive 'being-carried-away' and 'floaty' connotations of 'flow'. Undoubtedly, 'dynamic aliveness' is a modality of awareness very close to optimal performance but one that is *oriented towards compositional generation and organization*. As such, 'dynamic aliveness' can be viewed as a distinct expression or specific channelling of flow. In a nutshell, although all instances of 'dynamic aliveness' involve flow, not all flow experiences are 'dynamically alive' in the compositional sense. This is a distinction that, as a practitioner and as an observer of practitioners, I can recognize, precisely because of the different *phenomenological tones* involved. Improvisation provides valuable clues in this regard.

In their chapter on anticipation and improvisation in the *Handbook of Embodied Cognition and Sport Psychology* (Cappuccio 2019), psychiatrist Nelson Mauro Maldonato, psychobiologist Alberto Oliverio, and computer scientist Anna Esposito consider Csikszentmihalyi's flow from a neurocognitive outlook. They view it as:

a temporal interval during which a routine ability or a well-trained cognitive function operate without the interference of the explicit [conscious] system: this way of operating is characterized by a state of

162   *Performer Training for Actors and Athletes*

lesser activity of the prefrontal lobe, in such a way that the analytical capacities of the explicit system are temporarily "switched off" [Jeanne Nakamura in Csikszentmihalyi and Csikszentmihalyi 1988]. However, […] the condition of flow requires explicit attention in order to endure and, therefore, an extended status of flow requires the activation of the frontal neural network.

(Maldonato et al. 2019: 707–8)

In other words: a degree of low-level awareness remains even when the subject is fully immersed in a manner that disengages her explicit cognitive processing during an activity. The authors' account of improvisation (mainly with regard to music but also cross-referencing dance and sports like football) resonates with this understanding of flow, ascribing the ensuing minimal awareness to 'a sort of internal generator of thoughts and ideas, memories and images, that crop up spontaneously and often unexpectedly in the consciousness, [and that] is related to the so-called *default mode network*' (Maldonato et al. 2019: 710, emphasis in the original). Importantly, it is the activation of this network that compensates for the 'switching off' of conscious control.

This default mode network is reminiscent of another phenomenon noted earlier in the chapter: the *internal template* or subconscious *idealized sensorial image* that athletes acquire with extensive practice. I had suggested that this template functions as a fluid standard or *aesthetic* that measures and regulates (assesses and shapes) the execution of action. As such, this internal mechanism in endurance athletics was aligned with Zarrilli's 'aesthetic inner bodymind', with the latter marking a subtle embodied capacity that experienced actors and dancers cultivate through deep psychophysical processes.

Maldonato et al.'s 'internal generator of thoughts and ideas, memories and images' corresponds in part to what in everyday parlance goes by the general term of 'imagination', which the authors consider crucial in the forging of new pathways and connections (2019: 703). In this regard, the flow of images and associations that characterized 'dynamic aliveness' during the plastiques and *Tekhnē Sessions* improvisations, especially their lack of predetermination, resonate with the operational dynamics of such an 'internal generator'. They are also what drove the *compositional* dimension of the 'little' narratives and dramaturgies that emerged in the course of the improvisations.

An important aspect identified by Maldonato et al. corroborates, from a neurocognitive angle, the current chapter's emphasis on experience. It highlights the reasons *why* experience is essential for both 'peak performance'

Performance Through Experience 163

and 'efficacious improvisation'. Without extensive experience, Maldonato and colleagues argue that:

> there is no possibility of *high-level automatisms*, hence no opportunity to trigger the involuntary memory and, subsequently, no space for *enacting creative play through the imaginative exploration* of possible worlds. That is why expert performers show a more marked capacity for deactivating their selective attention, compared with budding musicians and non-musicians.
>
> (Maldonato et al. 2019: 710, emphasis added)

There is, indeed, a difference between the desirable automaticity of mastered technique and assimilated material that enables athletic and artistic inventiveness versus the deadening automation of mechanized behaviour that results in predictable patterns. This insight feeds directly into the paradoxical nature of the 'almost automatic yet highly focused state of consciousness' that typifies Csikszentmihalyi's flow experiences (1996: 110), a phenomenon that aligns well with the sensations of 'unfocused focus' or 'inverted distraction' in the above case studies of 'dynamic aliveness'. The inverse of this enabling automaticity is 'choking' in athletic performance (Chapter 2) and 'stage fright' in theatre (Chapter 4), where the excessive focused attention on oneself and on technique impairs one's performance.

Another key element that emerged in my experience of dynamic aliveness which finds some support in Maldonato et al.'s study concerns the dynamic of *solo* performance. Discussing group improvisation in music, the authors argue that 'the necessary harmonization of emerging materials, typical of a group performance, hinders the "turning off" of the prefrontal structures and, on the contrary, raises the level of conscious attention' (2019: 712–13). Similar conditions were found in team sports where the variables in play are considerably numerous and more complex than in a solo event. Indeed, an explicit endeavour to generate collective harmony in groups or dialogic synchronicity in duos becomes the equivalent of an 'internal focus' in individual performance (Chapter 1), with the consequence that one is always *self-consciously* (however *minimally*) playing 'catch up' to achieve and *maintain* that connection. Crucial to group performance is the ability to function as one without thinking about it, hence the requirement of an exceptional degree of mutual automaticity *as a base for creative solutions*. Due to the explicit goal-determined outcome in team sports (where you either score a point or not), such reciprocity is more evident when it lacks or fails than in aesthetic ensemble work. Such discrepancies in theatre or

164   *Performer Training for Actors and Athletes*

dance can be partly mitigated by shifting the attention elsewhere (e.g. through lighting, music, spatial positioning, costumes, or a prominence of individual actions).

The decisive role that improvisation plays in the *compositional* aspect of the flow states associated with 'dynamic aliveness' is foregrounded in the distinction that Maldonato et al. make between improvisers like jazz players and the 'performer of scores' (2019: 711). Such a differentiation recognizes the one being posited between the *specific flow* of 'dynamic aliveness' and *other flow* manifestations. Maldonato et al.'s distinction does not exclude the 'performer of scores' (i.e. the recitalist) from experiencing flow, especially if she is highly skilled and playing in solo conditions. In such cases, and as I tried to investigate in the First Movement of *Tekhnē Sessions* where improvisation was explored within a highly codified structure (Figure 6), although there is scope for improvisation, it occurs not so much with the form or design but with its enactment. That is, the performer is focused on *interpreting by following* a pre-existing structure for which she has prepared and trained in advance. This means that optimal and peak performances of scripted work *flow-through* existing channels rather than *flow-forge* new pathways through the inventiveness of improvisation. Again, this does not exclude the performer of scores from creativity or ingenuity during her interpretation, but it marks a different processing modality of embodied cognition.

Maldonato et al.'s discernment between improvisers and recitalists echoes the one made earlier between 'actor-creators' and 'actor-interpreters' (Murphy 2019a: 7), which resonates with Zarrilli's more general distinction between 'actor-as-maker' and 'actor-as-interpreter' (Zarrilli 2013: 7). It is not a coincidence that Lecoq's pedagogy, which epitomizes Murphy's actor-creator, is based on various modes of improvisation during training. Lecoq's *jeu* (playfulness) is at the core of his training, not only in terms of mask work and movement but also in the imagination of the 'mind' as exemplified through his mimodynamic approach. This applies in different ways to other physical practices. For example, apart from providing a solid technical formation, Grotowski's plastiques achieve their fuller potential during improvisation that, as we saw, transcend the technique to tap into an individual's memory resources and enable deeper modalities of performing. If in Maldonato et al. the emphasis is on the musician-improviser's 'perception of the specific possibilities and limitations offered by her instrument' (2019: 711), in aesthetic performance genres like physical theatre and dance, where the performer's 'instrument' *is* her own body, the felt perception of one's psychophysiological and technical capacities are decisive factors.

Notwithstanding the emphasis on improvisation as an important dynamic in training, the majority of actors from a Lecoq background, as

Performance Through Experience 165

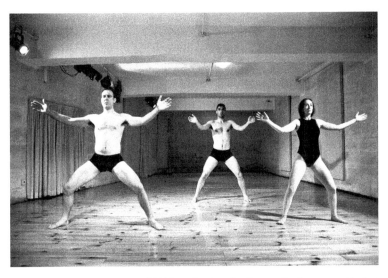

Figure 6 First Movement of *Tekhnē Sessions* by Icarus Performance Project (ActionBase Studio, Malta, 2004). Photo by Sandro Spina.

well as those who worked with other psychophysical practitioners like Grotowski and Barba, perform in highly structured productions. As such, they also *interpret* scores that – despite arising from improvisations and collective creation rather than from interpretations of written texts – end up *becoming* prescribed. Does this mean that these actor-creators become actor-interpreters of their work? This is a question worth unpacking, albeit briefly to round up the argument.

Whether as training or as performance, an improvisation practice puts the performer 'on the line' in the sense that it fosters and ingrains a capacity that 'anything can happen'. This is related to the phenomenon that Lecoq highlights in the context of neutral mask improvisation: 'to watch, to hear, to feel, to touch elementary things with the freshness of beginnings' (Lecoq [1997] 2002: 38; Camilleri 2020a: 30–3). It is in these defamiliarizing 'fresh' ways that improvisation-based practices are liberatory because they do not teach the mechanized automaticity of an actor's 'bag of tricks' (Whyman 2013: 1) but nurture, instead, an attitude of being and doing that is capable of coping even with highly structured scores.

The crucial difference that a deep practice of improvisation makes, then, resides with the *modality of inhabitation*. The embodied 'mind' of Maldonato et al.'s jazz player or of an actor-creator, accustomed to improvisation as

166   *Performer Training for Actors and Athletes*

they are, does not suddenly alter when reciting a prescribed score. On the contrary, that *embodiment adapts its inventiveness to its perceptually enacted reality*, hence the relevance of distinguishing between different modes of flow phenomenologies that the compositional dimension of 'dynamic aliveness' foregrounds in aesthetic and athletic contexts.

*

As the three chapters in Part II make evident, the various components in affective science's configuration of emotion episodes are discrete only in name because they overlap with and bleed into each other, sometimes even skipping their sequentiality.

And yet a componential approach to sensorial perception, emotional inflection, and actional outcome has provided a way of seeing the multi-layered connections and organicity that is connoted by the multivalent word 'feeling'.

This is of special relevance for somatic practices like the performing arts and sports that necessarily involve body–world relationalities which they *intensify* and *amplify* through deep and durational processes.

Conclusion

Along the *Via Athletae*

Setting the Scene

Writing from experience as a runner, sociologist Jacquelyn Allen Collinson's autoethnography on injury and rehabilitation (2005) brings together the major stands in this book, i.e. body, mind, and emotions as featured in 'Part I: Mind Games' and 'Part II: Heart Matters'. Her sports-inflected elaboration on the pioneering work of Arlie Russell Hochschild's sociology of emotions, specifically regarding the distinction between 'deep acting' and 'surface acting' in daily life, illuminates acting processes in aesthetic performance. In this light, Franco Ruffini's explanation of a quality of skilled behaviour that he associates with the 'reality' and consequent 'truth' of an action – *azione in vita* (action in life) – takes on different hues (1995: 54). Indeed, in the intersection between Allen Collinson's 'acting *in* life' and Ruffini's 'acting *as in* life', it is possible to correlate 'deep' and 'surface' behaviours with their real/true status. In view of the resonances traced in the Introduction between *azione in vita* and the proposal of *via athletae* ('way of the athlete'), it is appropriate to conclude this volume with a reconsideration of certain assumptions along with an appraisal of some implications for practice.

In Allen Collinson's account, deep acting corresponds with attempts 'to feel what we sense we ought to feel or want to feel' as distinct from 'the deliberate, contrived [...] outward display of emotions' of surface acting (2005: 233). Despite the overlying proximity of '*wanting* to feel' and '*deliberate* feeling', she argues that: 'Deep acting [...] produces a more "*genuine*" outward display via the generation of *actual* feeling that has been *self-induced* by the social actor. In surface acting the actor experiences the emotional display as put on, not "part of me" – in deep acting the actor *actually* experiences the emotions as *authentic*' (233, emphasis added). The difference, therefore, concerns the *connection* between feeling and its display, rather than the *how* that feeling was generated because, as shall be seen, both qualities can be predetermined and constructed. Furthermore, the 'genuine'

168 *Performer Training for Actors and Athletes*

display of 'actual' feelings and 'authentic' emotions sits well with the ethical dimension of 'truth' ascribed to Ruffini's functional *azione in vita*, as it does with Lecoq's 'economical' movement that reflects life and the biomechanical self (Lecoq [1987] 2006: 81).

The Introduction problematized the reality/truth status of actions by evoking Brendan Ingle's controversial incorporation of 'theatrical' non-boxing elements in his coaching for boxers. In the same vein, the reality/truth of actions can be also deconstructed by the 'self-inducing' quality of deep acting that presents a 'genuineness' and 'authenticity' that is *manufactured*. Does this engineered phenomenon make the action any less real or true? Reflections from theatre history, from Denis Diderot's eighteenth-century Paradox of the Actor (or the capacity of actors to display emotion without feeling it) to Konstantin Stanislavski's fusion of 'personal reality' with the role (Hodge 2010a: xix–xx; Benedetti 2000: 91), tell us that it does not matter as long as the manifested action–emotion is credible, irrespective of how it is achieved. However, the notion of a fabricated or constructed process does put a fly in the consecrating ointment of what supposedly constitutes 'real' and 'true' behaviour, rendering it anything but 'natural', 'pure', 'unmediated', or 'spontaneous'.

In the Introduction, the reality–truth nexus of *azione in vita* is situated within a *modality* of doing. Although 'modality' involves both *matter* and, especially, *manner* of doing, it could be understood as some kind of *frequency* or *wavelength* to which one attunes when performing. Such a 'wavelength of doing' recalls the case studies of Chapter 6 that deal with a *modality* of compositional 'dynamic aliveness' in aesthetic training and performance as well as in certain moments during long runs. Likewise, but in a different configuration, it is the *modality* or *wavelength* of Ingle's coaching that matters rather than the actual content, format, or patterns of that training. For a movement can be functional and economical but if it constitutes 'surface acting' it amounts to 'fabrication' in the sense of fake and forgery (Oxford English Dictionary). Conversely, it is possible for 'theatrical' and 'extravagant' movement to constitute 'deep acting' if it contributes to and is constitutive of holistic engagement, i.e. 'fabrication' in the sense of constructed or assembled by art, skill, or labour (Oxford English Dictionary).

In this scenario, Allen Collinson's downplaying *adjustment* of her feelings of relief (about recovering from injury) is judged as a compassionate gesture of 'genuine sympathy and support' for her running partner whose rehabilitation was not as advanced. Here, the regulation of the *experience* and *display* of emotions becomes constitutive of a 'method' of deep acting (2005: 233). A similar process applies to the case of emotion modulation in Chapter 5 concerning the volitional smiling to counter the negative impact of exertion during intensity running, thus conditioning an athlete's sensorial

Conclusion: Along the Via Athletae   169

and emotional feelings (Brick et al. 2018). Likewise with the positive effects of self-talk in endurance performance (Blanchfield et al. 2014). All these instances mark conscious self-induced behaviour, and therefore *manufactured processes* that result in credible actions that are physiologically 'real' and perceived/experienced (by doer and other) as emotionally 'true'. In the words of Chapter 5, the 'outer' physical *simulation* (e.g. smiling and positive self-talk) leads to the 'internal' emotional *stimulation* of those states (cf. Gallagher and Gallagher 2020: 783–6). Chapter 5's distinction between 'smiling *to feel* happy' and 'smiling *because I feel* happy' is also relevant to Allen Collinson's subdued feelings of relief and other forms of quotidian deep acting. As per Chapter 6's title, it becomes a question of 'putting on an act', a performance that ends up, literally, *acting upon oneself*. This kind of work upon the self brings me to *via athletae*, a journey of self-transformation through training, in sports and aesthetic performance but also in daily life.

As presented in the Introduction, *via athletae* marks a way of being 'true' to one's bodyworld, thus signalling a modality of doing that is also an ethical stance in its relational commitment. In material terms, this *corporeal truth* to the *situating reality* is manifested in the *affordances* that arise in the interactive specificities between bodies and world. These affordances emerge in the individual's perception as much as they exist in the situating environment. As such, 'affordances' are always already *bodyworld affordances* that correspond to a practitioner's skill level (e.g. Araújo et al. 2019: 567–8), which means that they can be worked upon and enhanced. The actualization of one's bodyworld affordances in *azione in vita* (*of* one's body and *of* the surrounding environment) makes *via athletae* a quest of the self that, through training, lends itself to a re-making of the self.

What sets *via athletae* apart from other ways of being is the accent on physical engagement as an intensified encounter with the world's materiality. More precisely, it is the *modality* of that intensity and engagement, specifically its *autotelic playfulness* and *inherent competitiveness* (in the etymological sense of 'flying with' and as it overlaps with Georges Hébert's *auto émulation*), which distinguishes it from related practices. In comparison, Artaud's total theatre comes across as too self-annihilatory in the quest for self-discovery and its resultant manifestation on stage. Likewise, Grotowski's poor theatre appears too sacrificially 'Christ-like', serious and heavy with the weight of the world on one's shoulders to be 'playful', with the quest of the self being that of salvation, from oneself and for the world. Conversely, Lecoq's mime is relatively too light in its neutral mask tonalities and comedic potential, and too light weight in its technical codification, especially when compared to Decroux's corporeal mime, which in turn is closer to Grotowski's spirit. Despite the reductive sketchiness of these comparisons, their broad

170   *Performer Training for Actors and Athletes*

brushstrokes serve to situate-by-association the novel element that is *via athletae* in a constellation of known practices, thus identifying what is distinctive about it. Of course, all the above and similar psychophysical approaches are extremely effective in and beyond the theatre. Moreover, given the *modality* or 'wavelength' of engagement, they can serve as *via athletae* in their own right.

As observed in the preceding chapters, the commitment associated with *via athletae* is pushed to extremes in endurance sports. It bears repeating that the physicality of such engagement includes the mental as an irreducible dimension. Matt Fitzgerald articulates the point in terms of a 'mental fitness' that is as specific to the individual as an optimal running economy (2016: 261–2). From the perspective of *via athletae*, the uniqueness Fitzgerald identifies is that of one's bodyworld affordances, which include psychophysical capacities. Tellingly, Fitzgerald relates these capacities to 'being oneself', which again underscores a quest or training of the self to improve that 'individual formula' (2016: 264), hence the individual process of *via athletae* that borders also on the autodidactic or even, in apprenticeship models, guided autodidacticism (Camilleri 2015a: 22–3).

'Being oneself' *at the same time as* improving and changing that self through psychosomatic engagement marks a *via* like the one being proposed here. In this sense, Decroux's '*via positiva*' (Ingemar Lindh's term for the technical intricacy of corporeal mime; 1995: 66) and Grotowski's *via negativa* (the eradication of psychophysical obstacles) can both contribute to or constitute a *via athletae*. In a different dimension, even so-called 'mindless' practices like running on a treadmill while watching a screen in a gym (Zarrilli 2009: 30) or high intensity aerobics can contribute to (but rarely constitute on their own) a *via athletae if* incorporated within a milieu whose overarching *modality* conforms to what has been identified as the 'corporeal truth to the situating reality that affordances make manifest' (e.g. in the case of a running practice, *if* inserted within the context of weekly speed, steady, recovery, hill, and long runs).

Practise What You Preach

The final part of the Conclusion compiles some key aspects from the preceding chapters that occur in skilled practices but whose playful and competitive engagement can be aligned with *via athletae*. The way of being *athletae* is not a prescribed or prescribing method but a *modality of habitation*, hence the emphasis on the structures and qualities that require the actualization of being 'lived in'.

Conclusion: Along the Via Athletae   171

The 'Along the *Via Athletae*' list below is preceded by an exercise that has been evolving in my physical theatre practice since the mid-1990s, initially as part of a personal and group process, subsequently according to coaching exigencies within Icarus Performance Project, intensive workshops, and university modules. It characterizes various aspects of aesthetic performance training, thus offering the possibility of a habitational mode conducive to *via athletae*, especially considering that it was designed for the purpose of playfully enabling compositional improvisation (see also Chapter 6). Apart from its inherent appeal as a training exercise, it illuminates certain elements in the *via athletae* list that follows it. Ideally, the exercise, list, and commentary should be presented side-by-side but the linear imperatives of writing and printing offer other affordances.

The Sphere Exercise

The Sphere Exercise is an effective way of working on *awareness* within a *physical* and *imaginative* context, thus aiming to enhance all three dimensions holistically. The exercise develops an all-round capacity to move in different directions and levels: in front of, behind, either side of, above, and below oneself, plus various combinations of these. Consequently, I sometimes refer to '360-degree sphere awareness' when transmitting the exercise. Furthermore, the improved ability 'to move' sensitizes also the capacity 'to be moved by', thus also impacting the affective dimension.

Starting Points

- The *quality of engagement* in every step of the exercise is essential. Focus on fulfilling each task.
- The *duration of every layer* in the Sphere Exercise is relative to one's mastery. In the early phases of learning, substantial time is dedicated to each step before progressing to the next one. For example, circa 20 minutes per layer for three sessions a week until a degree of fluency is achieved. When mastered, the entire exercise can take 20 minutes in total.
- Adopting a horse-riding stance, with the soles of the feet rooted to the floor and a low + reactive centre of gravity for a steady yet flexible base, start by *imagining* that you are inhabiting a sphere, i.e. a 360-degree active space. Look around you and *see* (visualize) the sphere.

172   *Performer Training for Actors and Athletes*

Base Layer (foundational level of the exercise)

- The first task is to *touch, with the tip of a finger, the extreme edges* (or the 'extremities') of the sphere, thus fully engaging your body as you stretch to your limits. Fill *evenly* the 360-degree space around you with imaginary spots as you touch the sphere.
- Proceed to *extending these spots into lines of different lengths*, e.g. from 5 cm-long-lines to 50 cm to 1 metre. Your sphere is now filling up with imaginary lines of different lengths. 'Imaginatively concretize' the lines with specific thicknesses and colours, making them 'real' by your action–perception.
- Do the same with the other extremities in the sphere: *the proximities*, i.e. the areas closest to (without actually touching) your body.
- Explore different *dynamics of speed* (from very fast to fast to normal to slow to very slow) *and effort* (from very light to light to normal to heavy to very heavy), eventually – when mastered – bringing all aspects together in different combinations for every action (e.g. front + below + very light + slow).
- For a more embodied *felt perception* of speed and effort I refer to the speed spectrum as '*the urgencies*' (e.g. from 'not urgent at all' to 'late for an appointment' to 'being chased by someone in the dark') and the effort range as '*the resistances*' (e.g. moving in air, in water, in stone, or in steel), hence fusing further the connection between movement and imagination via intentionality.

Additional Layers (developing the Base Layer)

- *Engaging Different Parts of the Body.* Use different parts of the body to inject spots and draw lines in the sphere. For example, start with the joints in your hands and arms, moving from fingertips to knuckles, to wrists, to elbows, to shoulders. Even non-joint areas like the sides of individual fingers and the palms or backs of hands can be sensitized in this way, physically and imaginatively, but potentially also emotionally in other layers of the exercise.
- *Moving in Space.* Move in the space by adopting different parts of the leg (knees, heels, toes, sides of the feet, etc.) to draw spots and lines of different lengths, thicknesses, and colours. Though your feet are no longer rooted to the floor in this layer, you can now move in the space while still being *grounded*.
- *Eye Work.* During the initial stages of working on the Base Layer, *look at* the spots or lines that you produce. Eventually, *look at something*

Conclusion: Along the Via Athletae   173

else in the space, away from what you are doing. Such a move changes 'everything' for you as doer (and for observers of your work) because it opens your actions to yet another direction, this time beyond the sphere, beyond you, making your behaviour inherently and explicitly 'dramatic' in embodying a dialogue or conflict with an 'other'. This marks a key aspect of the Sphere Exercise because engaging the eyes in this way enables you to work on *multiple intentions* simultaneously: looking at a specific spot in the space while drawing a line in a different direction, all the time with feet rooted or moving in (thus 'pointing at') yet another direction.

- *The Face.* Deploy different parts of your face and head to draw spots and lines: use the tip of your nose or tongue, your chin or cheeks, eyebrows, ears, throat, nape, etc. You can even activate your eyes in this manner. Be imaginative and playful, explore different points. This can be an effective way of working on facial expressions without resorting to (i.e. *starting from*) emotions. And yet the work *can be* emotional, potentially generating feelings in the doer (and observer) through socio-cultural and body memory.

Advanced Layers (incorporating devising possibilities)

- *Designing Stories.* Create different patterns and shapes (including letters of the alphabet and numbers) with the spots and lines, thus adding a layer of compositional and narrative organization that can be repeated and recalled.
- *Multiple Lines.* Introduce additional action points for spots and lines, i.e. you can have two (or more) lines going on simultaneously, with contrasting or resonating 'urgencies' and/or 'resistances'. This layer offers various possibilities of dramatic/dialogic activity, including 'ignoring' one of the lines, perhaps to pick it up later, thus remaining aware of it without physically pursuing it, once again exercising a complex intentionality.
- *Co-Sphere.* Work with a partner, starting back-to-back, where the two of you alternate in drawing spots and lines in the combined spaces of your spheres. (I have utilized and developed this layer as a separate exercise in its own right as a devising and rehearsal strategy involving two or more performers.)
- *Voice & Text.* Use the voice and/or deliver an improvised or memorized text during, after, or even *instead* of drawing a spot or a line. Combined with 'co-sphere' partner work this has considerable dramatic and improvisatory potential.

174   *Performer Training for Actors and Athletes*

Final Layer (compositional structures *towards* and *as* performance)

- The final stage of the Sphere Exercise is to *improvise* with all the above sensitized areas and dynamics of the body, first technically (where one can recognize the technique of imaginary spots and lines) and then beyond-technically (where the movements are closer to everyday actions, but which are driven by the internal logic of spots, lines, and the sphere). An example of the latter may include the *manifested action* of picking up an object from the floor or smoking a cigarette or leaping over an obstacle while saying a text, but the *internal logic* of the movement is that of assimilated spots and lines. Figure 1 and Figure 4 in Chapter 6 display instances of performance material influenced by the Sphere Exercise, with Figure 4 also exemplifying the layer of Multiple Lines.
- Organize your improvisation into an *overarching structure* that has a beginning, middle, and an end. The structure does not need to be either predetermined or logical, e.g. it can start in one corner of the room and end in another, or you can remain in the same spot throughout.

Note

The Sphere Exercise is loosely inspired by the evocation of space in Rudolf Laban's kinesphere, the fragmentation/articulation of the body in Jerzy Grotowski's plastiques, and Ingemar Lindh's practice of improvisation as performance. An earlier barebones version of the exercise was the so-called 'Thread Work' by John J. Schranz, director of Groups for Human Encounter. Thread Work consisted of 'threading silk lines in the space' by means of a thumb-and-index-finger grip and then by other parts of the body. The later elaborations were by me, some while still working with Schranz and others after I set up Icarus Performance Project. Some aspects of the Sphere Exercise feature in the 'Awareness' short video of *Physical Actor Training – An Online A–Z* (Allain et al. 2018).

Along the *Via Athletae*: List and Commentary

'Along the *Via Athletae*' gathers elements from this book that can be aligned with a psychophysical *modality* of performing inspired by athletic activity. While the first two categories in the list refer to conditions of possibility

Conclusion: Along the Via Athletae   175

that also apply to other practices and ways of being, the third and fourth provide a sense of what a *via athletae* might entail. To counter the inevitable reductiveness of a list, brackets after an item indicate the main chapter where it is discussed in more detail. The relevant items can also be referenced in the Index for further information.

1. **Affordances of Practitioner Body–World Assemblages** [Introduction]. Including:
   a. an individual's psychophysical traits and related capacities, such as physical, vocal, and sensory characteristics like height and weight as well as quality of vision and hearing, speed and propensities of cognitive processing, pain threshold, and memory retention;
   b. environmental features as they concern indoor or outdoor settings and their respective ambient and climate conditions;
   c. equipment, including clothing, technology, and infrastructure that mediate the body–world interaction by operating on the affordances of the body (e.g. footwear that conditions one's movement) and of the world (e.g. climate controlled systems and road infrastructure).

Commentary

A personal example of *affordances* concerns my short-sightedness, which is corrected by the use of glasses in daily life and when leading practical sessions, including when transmitting the Sphere Exercise. However, I prefer not to wear glasses when training on my own or performing because that short-sightedness paradoxically assists my holistic focus in at least two ways:

   i. No aspect of my awareness, however minuscule, is (pre)occupied with the probability of the glasses slipping down my nose or of banging them against my face during high energy movement sequences. This means that my attention (see No. 2 in the List) has a lower probability of triggering an internal focus with the attendant risks of 'choking' or hindering optimal flow.
   ii. The blurred eyesight enhances my other senses, not only by compensation but by transforming the impairment into an advantage due to the increased *physical* sense of *being present*. I often experience this organic alertness and readiness as some kind of primordial survival mode that heightens my perception during aesthetic performance activity.

Although practically every aspect of human training and performance can be subsumed under assemblages and affordances, including their resultant actualized status as socio-cultural actants (hence the 3As of bodyworld), it is possible to fine-tune the analysis with reference to aesthetic and athletic practices. In this regard, the categorizing impulse of sports science, especially as covered in Chapters 1 and 2, can be adapted for a nuanced appreciation of *attentional focus*.

2. **Attentional Focus** [Chapter 1, Chapter 2; Brick et al. 2014; Wulf 2013]. Including:
   a. internal sensory monitoring, regarding breathing, heart rate, muscle soreness, fatigue, etc.;
   b. outward monitoring as relevant to ongoing action, e.g. cues in aesthetic performance, route markers and other signage in a competitive event, and information made available by sports watches (like distance covered and pace);
   c. internal or proximal focus, i.e. on a specific muscle or body movement whilst executing an action;
   d. external or distal focus, i.e. on the movement effect, an implement deployed, or the environment more widely;
   e. active distraction, e.g. intentional tasks not related to the activity (like mentally working out a mathematical sum), busy urban streets, conversation with a partner, audience chatter;
   f. involuntary distraction, e.g. attractive scenery, scanning the audience while performing, daydreaming.

Commentary

The 'extremities' and 'proximities' in the Sphere Exercise do not correspond respectively to 'external' or 'internal' focus because the emphasis is on the imaginary spots and lines rather than on the body part generating them. More accurately, the 'extremities' and 'proximities' enact the range of distal relations *within* the practitioner's 'sphere' of psychophysical influence. As such they *exercise* attentional focus in a manner that 'stretches' its flexibility as if it were another muscle.

The Eye Work layer in the same exercise offers another possibility of engaging an external focus by directing attention *away from* one's movements towards a point beyond the sphere, in the process minimizing the likelihood of the self-conscious internal focus that tends to trigger choking and stage fright (see Chapter 2 and Chapter 4).

Conclusion: Along the Via Athletae   177

3. **Behavioural Adaptations**. Including:
   a. physiological ('recessive') regulation [Chapter 3];
   b. volitional (psycho/physical) adjustment, mainly as a result of internal sensory monitoring and as conditioned by training (e.g. adjustment of breathing pattern to reduce heart rate), also as manifested via action readiness (e.g. muscular activation in preparation for specific actions) [Chapter 4];
   c. emotion modulation via enactment of desired state (e.g. smiling, frowning, self-talk) or evocation of specific memories/images, including to condition perception of effort [Chapter 5].

Commentary

Although qualities of the phenomenologically recessive 'visceral' body (Zarrilli 2009: 52–5) are hard to regulate, especially of the deeper (non-conscious) type discussed in Chapter 3 that arise when the body is pushed to the limit, certain aspects can be intervened upon indirectly. Examples of such adjustments include modifying breathing patterns to calm the heart rate as well as focused imagination and positive self-talk to minimize the risk or overcome moments of 'choking' and stage fright.

A case in point of behavioural adaptation involves the Face layer of the Sphere Exercise, which indirectly operates on the modulation of emotion through the enactment of facial expressions as discussed in Chapter 5 during running. The stretching and patterning of the facial muscles during this stage of the Sphere Exercise tend to organically activate associations that accompany the same facial configurations of certain emotional states in daily life. As argued earlier, the 'constructed' *simulation* of an outer reality becomes conducive to the 'truthful' *stimulation* of an inner state. The difference in the Sphere Exercise is that the practitioner does not will, desire, or otherwise predetermine the facial simulation because she is operating according to the intentionality of drawing dots-and-lines-in-space.

Within this context, the manifestation of 'true' emotion in 'real' physical action has the potential of emerging (of leaking out) before it is phenomenologically and cognitively processed by the practitioner. As discussed in Chapter 4, perception necessarily involves filtering, even before it is recognized or evaluated as such. It is precisely this borderline non-/awareness of perception that spells its *playful* value for *via athletae* and ultimately for theatrical performance. Similar to Stanislavski's work on physical actions, which he found more reliable than the volatility of deploying emotions on stage night after night, the Face layer of the

178 Performer Training for Actors and Athletes

Sphere Exercise seeks to stimulate the practitioner's *azione in vita*, exactly by retaining the focus on the intentionality and physicality of her doing. Trained in this way, the actor – like the elite athlete – taps into the liberatory and creative automaticity (as distinct from the mechanized automaticity of merely repeated behaviour) that allows her to 'live' the role 'functionally' and 'economically' *as if* in daily life.

In the modification of behaviour, whether consciously or otherwise, the role of technique as a *way of doing* is foregrounded. In the current context, *via athletae* marks a modality or frequency of such technique-conditioned doing as manifested in *performance dynamics*.

4. Performance Dynamics
    a. pacing [Chapter 3];
    b. play and competitive 'flying with' [Introduction];
    c. optimal flow [Chapter 2];
    d. compositional improvisation [Chapter 6].

Commentary

Even more than *Behavioural Adaptations*, the category of *Performance Dynamics* is the main distinctive feature of a *via athletae* practice.

Pacing marks *via athletae*'s overarching *organizational impetus in performance*. It involves (1) *macro structures* like planning and strategy that are enabled and concretized by (2) *middle level mechanisms* like method and technique that are driven and inhabited by (3) *grassroots dynamics and textures*, including those of 'playful competitiveness'. Although in this understanding of pacing the intermediate role of technique is essential for the actualization of strategy and scores, it is precisely the *inhabited (actualized) dynamics of doing* that determine the *modality* of a performance event. In thus bringing together 'technique assimilation' and 'preparation planning' while not being either *because it cannot be enacted except in performance*, pacing epitomizes the *modality of habitation*. This applies also to Chapter 3's *aesthetic pacing* that concerns the performed unfolding of all levels of a theatre score or dance choreography.

Understood principally as the *management* of one's resources *in* performance, pacing is the manifested culmination of a process that begins *before* an aesthetic or athletic event and that continues *after* it finishes until the next iteration. The longer trajectory of pacing that spans multiple events (e.g. a theatre season or a sports championship), includes the ongoing training and assessment of one's capacities as well as the specific planning and organization for the individual performances or competitions. Set against

Conclusion: Along the Via Athletae   179

this background, 'pacing', especially as demonstrated in the one-step-after-another simplicity of long-distance running, paints a fuller picture of the dynamics involved. Mihaly Csikszentmihalyi's 'optimal flow' (Chapter 2) and my notion of 'dynamic aliveness' during compositional improvisation (Chapter 6) are both phenomenological states that at once manifest and influence particular *experiences of pacing*. Although flow and compositional aliveness are not exclusive to *via athletae*, their conditions of possibility and resultant affordances facilitate the modality. As such, pacing offers a key to *via athletae*.

Chapter 2's discussion of epistemic actions (in aesthetic performance) and secondary/dual tasks (in sports) underlines specific dynamics that contribute to pacing modalities. In brief, epistemic behaviour refers to actions that accomplish an objective in an indirect manner, thus also offering a nuanced perspective on intentionality. Rebecca Loukes has proposed considering Stanislavski's work on physical actions as 'epistemic' because of its ulterior objective/intention of developing a character (Loukes 2013: 242). Dual tasks usually involve an additional focus unrelated to the main action, e.g. a footballer concentrating on a specific section of the environment while taking a penalty kick, with the ultimate intention of avoiding an internal focus that can trigger choking (Wulf and Lewthwaite 2010: 93–5; Chapter 2). In this regard, and in different ways, both instances overlap with *active* or *volitional* distraction, again signalling a complex and multi-directional connection between intentionality and action.

The indirect dynamics of epistemic actions and dual tasks have a deeper significance than first meets the eye. In resisting the shortest path to an objective, they incarnate a *method* and an *ethos* based on an artist's or athlete's *processual self-organizing performance*, thus resonating with a *self-pacing* that transcends mere mechanical execution or reproduction. Such indirect dynamics, which share nothing with elaboration for its own sake, feature in other guises in aesthetic and athlete practices, including in the Multiple Lines layer of the Sphere Exercise and in cross-training in sports. Similarly, a crucial principle in Ingemar Lindh's practice was that of *alternation* (Camilleri 2008b: 439–40), which sought to combat the risk of 'mechanical and monotonous' modalities when continuously repeating movement to learn new material or when the material has been completely mastered. This is where the 'surprising oneself' of *alternation* comes in:

> I work on an action, I abandon it and direct myself to something else. Then, when I return to my first action, I do so from a completely different angle. In this way I find myself in a new situation and will have to grasp its substance and content immediately. The mechanical repetition of an

180   *Performer Training for Actors and Athletes*

action is not at all difficult but it kills the *vitality* in a gesture. One should reach such a profound knowledge of one's materials not only to be able to execute them, but also to catch them in *flight* at any moment.

(Lindh 2010: 35, emphasis added)

Lindh's choice of words is highly pertinent in echoing the actional *vitality* of the actor who *flies* (see Introduction), in the process underlining the imperative of *doing* that Ruffini associates with intentionality in life.

The Final Layer improvisation of the Sphere Exercise can be deployed for the purposes of retaining the 'vitality' of one's rehearsal and performance work. I refer specifically to the *inhabitation* of a performance score or choreography via the subterranean modality of spots and lines. Although the score remains (externally) the same, internally one can be moved (physically and emotionally) by the ever-vibrant task of developing and connecting lines that are always *compositionally* different; hence epitomizing and *living* the instruction to do *as if* for the first time.

The vibrancy or 'dynamic aliveness' that accompanies the Final Layer of the Sphere Exercise recalls a dramaturgical and performance strategy by Eugenio Barba for an actor to have a secret character in addition to her explicit performance role. As Odin Teatret actor Roberta Carreri recounts:

> Eugenio compared these two characters to the two horses used in battle by warriors of a tribe who fought against Alexander the Great. The warrior would utilise the two horses to conceal himself in the course of a battle, to bounce from one to the other with the aim of confusing the enemy, and to have at least one with which to return to camp. The secret character helps the actor to jump between two identities, thus avoiding the risk of giving a two-dimensional image of the explicit character. A *strategy*, therefore, aimed at avoiding the pitfall of clichés. If an actor does not manage to give shape to their explicit character, they can always fall back on the secret one for inspiration.
>
> (Carreri 2014: 98–9, Carreri 2003: 46, emphasis added)

Again, the choice of words is revealing in evoking a 'strategy' that aligns well with the concept of *dramaturgical (i.e. aesthetic) pacing*, especially when considering Barba's equine image of lasting the distance. If Lindh's *alternation* occurs mainly at the level of training or rehearsing, Barba's 'alternation' of horses/characters takes place at the level of dramaturgy and performance. Both instances reflect the broader trajectory that can be associated with

Conclusion: Along the Via Athletae   181

pacing as an organization (a planning and a management) of resources that stretches before and beyond the manifested activity in an event.

*

'Along the *Via Athletae*' does not specify a route but a journey, hence the necessity of pacing that is 'true' to the 'reality' of one's embodiment, irrespective of whether that involves running a marathon or playing a football match, or performing a realist character or a movement score.

The trained and constructed status of *skilled behaviour* that characterizes *via athletae* is not exclusive to performing artists and athletes. On the contrary, as a group of cognitive and sports scientists argue, one can see skilled behaviour also in daily life: 'We walk efficiently and effectively from place to place, effortlessly avoiding obstacles and preserving our balance. [...] *Skilled performance is the rule, not the exception*' (Wilson et al. 2019: 581, emphasis added).

The rule, not the exception. It is also in this sense, then, that skilled behaviour in aesthetic and athletic performance is 'real', precisely because it *reflects* and *is* what we do in daily life. The quality of *azione in vita* on stage and in sports constitutes what we tautologically practise in daily life. And when, like John Hockey's runners (Chapter 6), our trained and assembled 'form' *feels as if* we are 'flying along', then we are indeed dynamically alive along the *via athletae*.

References

Adam, Hajo, and Adam D. Galinsky. 2012. 'Enclothed Cognition', *Journal of Experimental Social Psychology*, 48 (4): 918–25.

Allain, Paul. 1997. *Gardzienice: Polish Theatre in Transition* (London: Routledge).

Allain, Paul. 2016. 'Thick Description/Thin Lines: Writing about Process in Contemporary Performance', *Contemporary Theatre Review*, 26 (4): 485–95.

Allain, Paul, Stacie Lee Bennett, and Frank Camilleri. 2018. *PATAZ: Physical Actor Training – An Online A–Z* (Drama Online, Bloomsbury). https://www.dramaonlinelibrary.com/physical-actor-training (accessed 24 August 2022).

Allen Collinson, Jacquelyn. 2005. 'Emotions, Interaction and the Injured Sporting Body', *International Review for the Sociology of Sport*, 40 (2): 221–40.

Aquilina, Stefan. 2013. 'Stanislavski and the Tactical Potential of Everyday Images', *Theatre Research International*, 38 (3): 229–39.

Aquilina, Stefan. 2016. 'As Simple but as Complex as Everyday Cooking: Stanislavski's Use of Physical Action in the Recreation of Nature', *Stanislavski Studies*, 4 (2): 111–24.

Araújo, Duarte, Keith Davids, and Patrick McGivern. 2019. 'The Irreducible Embeddedness of Action Choice in Sport', in Massimiliano L. Cappuccio (ed.), *Handbook of Embodied Cognition and Sport Psychology* (Cambridge, MA: MIT Press), pp. 537–55.

Araújo, Duarte, Matt Dicks, and Keith Davids. 2019. 'Selecting among Affordances: A Basis for Channeling Expertise', in Massimiliano L. Cappuccio (ed.), *Handbook of Embodied Cognition and Sport Psychology* (Cambridge, MA: MIT Press), pp. 557–80.

Artaud, Antonin. [1964] 2010. *The Theatre and Its Double*, rev., trans. by Victor Corti (Richmond: Alma Classics).

Baggio, Roberto. 1996. 'Baggio Apre Un Centro Buddista', *La Repubblica* (in Italian). 15 May. https://ricerca.repubblica.it/repubblica/archivio/repubblica/1996/05/15/baggio-apre-un-centro-buddista.html (accessed 24 August 2022).

Baker, Joseph, and Damian Farrow (eds). 2015. *Routledge Handbook of Sport Expertise* (London: Routledge).

Barad, Karen. 2007. *Meeting the Universe Halfway: Quantum Physics and the Entanglement of Matter and Meaning* (Durham, NC: Duke University Press).

Barba, Eugenio. [1993] 1995. *The Paper Canoe: A Guide to Theatre Anthropology*, trans. by Richard Fowler (London: Routledge).

Barba, Eugenio. 2010. *On Directing and Dramaturgy: Burning the House*, trans. by Judy Barba (London: Routledge).

References

Barba, Eugenio. 2021. 'The Two Lungs of the Actor: Introduction to Ana Correa's Work Demonstration', *Journal of Theatre Anthropology*, 1: 223–4.

Barba, Eugenio, and Nicola Savarese (eds). 2006. *A Dictionary of Theatre Anthropology: The Secret Art of the Performer*, 2nd edn (London: Routledge).

Barrett, Estelle, and Barbara Bolt (eds). 2009. *Practice as Research: Approaches to Creative Arts Enquiry* (London: I.B. Tauris).

Bauer, Patricia. 2018. 'Parkour (discipline of movement)', *Encyclopedia Britannica*. https://www.britannica.com/sports/parkour (accessed 24 August 2022).

Bay, Howard, Clive Barker, and George C. Izenour. 2021. 'Theatre (building)', *Encyclopedia Britannica*. https://www.britannica.com/art/theater-building (accessed 24 August 2022).

Benedetti, Jean. 2000. *Stanislavski: An Introduction* (London: Routledge).

Bennett, Jane. 2010. *Vibrant Matter: A Political Ecology of Things* (Durham, NC: Duke University Press).

Blanchfield, Anthony W., James Hardy, Helma Majella de Morree, Walter Staiano, and Samuele M. Marcora. 2014. 'Talking Yourself out of Exhaustion: The Effects of Self-talk on Endurance Performance', *Medicine & Science in Sports & Exercise*, 46 (5): 998–1007.

Borg, Gunnar. 1982. 'Psychophysical Bases of Perceived Exertion', *Medicine and Science in Sports and Exercise*, 14 (5): 377–81.

Borg, Gunnar. 1998. *Borg's Perceived Exertion and Pain Scales* (Champaign, IL: Human Kinetics).

Bragaru, Mihai, Rienk Dekker, and Jan H. B. Geertzen. 2012. 'Sport Prostheses and Prosthetic Adaptations for the Upper and Lower Limb Amputees: An Overview of Peer Reviewed Literature', *Prosthetics and Orthotics International*, 36 (3): 290–6.

Bramble, Dennis M., and Daniel E. Lieberman. 2004. 'Endurance Running and the Evolution of *Homo*', *Nature*, 432 (7015): 345–52.

Breitwieser, Sabine (ed.). 2014. *Simone Forti – Thinking with the Body* (Munich: Hirmer Verlag).

Brick, Noel, Tadhg MacIntyre, and Mark Campbell. 2014. 'Attentional Focus in Endurance Activity: New Paradigms and Future Directions', *International Review of Sport and Exercise Psychology*, 7 (1): 106–34.

Brick, Noel E., Megan J. McElhinney, and Richard S. Metcalfe. 2018. 'The Effects of Facial Expression and Relaxation Cues on Movement Economy, Physiological, and Perceptual Responses during Running', *Psychology of Sport and Exercise*, 34, 20–8.

Brietzke, Cayque, Paulo Estevao Franco-Alvarenga, Helio Jose Coelho-Junior, Rodrigo Silveira, Ricardo Yukio Asano, and Flavio Oliveira Pires. 2019. 'Effects of Carbohydrate Mouth Rinse on Cycling Time Trial Performance: A Systematic Review and Meta-Analysis', *Sports Medicine*, 49: 57–66.

Britton, John. 2010. 'The Pursuit of Pleasure', *Theatre, Dance and Performance Training*, 1 (1): 36–54.

184 References

Brown, Bryan. 2019. *A History of the Theatre Laboratory* (London: Routledge).

Calatayud, Joaquin, Jonas Vinstrup, Markus Due Jakobsen, Emil Sundstrup, Mikkel Brandt, Kenneth Jay, Juan Carlos Colado, and Lars Louis Andersen. 2016. 'Importance of Mind-Muscle Connection during Progressive Resistance Training', *European Journal of Applied Physiology*, 116: 527–33.

Calatayud, Joaquin, Jonas Vinstrup, Markus D. Jakobsen, Emil Sundstrup, Juan Carlos Colado, and Lars Louis Andersen. 2017. 'Mind-Muscle Connection Training Principle: Influence of Muscle Strength and Training Experience during a Pushing Movement', *European Journal of Applied Physiology*, 117: 1445–53.

Camilleri, Frank (ed.). 2004. *The Second Phase* (Malta: Icarus Performance Project).

Camilleri, Frank. 2008a. 'Collective Improvisation: The Practice and Vision of Ingemar Lindh', *TDR/The Drama Review*, 52 (1): 82–97.

Camilleri, Frank. 2008b. '"To Push the Actor-Training to Its Extreme": Training Process in Ingemar Lindh's Practice of Collective Improvisation', *Contemporary Theatre Review*, 18 (4): 425–41.

Camilleri, Frank. 2008c. 'Hospitality and the Ethics of Improvisation in the Work of Ingemar Lindh', *New Theatre Quarterly*, 24 (3): 246–59.

Camilleri, Frank. 2009. 'Of Pounds of Flesh and Trojan Horses: Performer Training in the Twenty-first Century', *Performance Research*, 14 (2): 26–34.

Camilleri, Frank. 2010. 'Tekhnē Sessions: Investigating Dynamic Aliveness in the Actor's Work', *Theatre, Dance and Performance Training*, 1 (2): 157–71.

Camilleri, Frank. 2011. 'Of Crossroads and Undercurrents: Ingemar Lindh's Practice of Collective Improvisation and Jerzy Grotowski', *New Theatre Quarterly*, 27 (4): 299–312.

Camilleri, Frank. 2013a. 'Between Laboratory and Institution: Practice as Research in No Man's Land', *TDR/The Drama Review*, 57 (1): 152–66.

Camilleri, Frank. 2013b. 'Making Visible the Invisible: Ingemar Lindh's Practice of Collective Improvisation and Étienne Decroux', *Contemporary Theatre Review*, 23 (3): 390–402.

Camilleri, Frank. 2013c. 'Yours Neutrally, Habitational Action: Performance between Theatre and Dance', *New Theatre Quarterly*, 29 (3): 247–63.

Camilleri, Frank. 2013d. 'Habitational Action: Beyond Inner and Outer Action', *Theatre, Dance and Performance Training*, 4 (1): 30–51.

Camilleri, Frank. 2015a. 'Towards the Study of Actor Training in an Age of Globalised Digital Technology', *Theatre, Dance and Performance Training*, 6 (1): 16–29.

Camilleri, Frank. 2015b. 'Of Hybrids and the Posthuman: Performer Training in the 21st Century', *TDR/The Drama Review*, 59 (3): 108–22.

Camilleri, Frank. 2017. 'Inverting the Formula: Devising through Adaptation', *New Theatre Quarterly*, 33 (3): 240–53.

Camilleri, Frank. 2018a. 'On Habit and Performer Training', *Theatre, Dance and Performance Training*, 9 (1): 36–52.

References

Camilleri, Frank. 2018b. 'Clues on *Technē*', *Performance Research*, 23 (4): 308–12.

Camilleri, Frank. 2019. *Performer Training Reconfigured: Post-psychophysical Perspectives for the Twenty-first Century* (London: Bloomsbury).

Camilleri, Frank. 2020a. 'From Bodymind to Bodyworld: The Case of Mask Work as a Training for the Senses', *Theatre, Dance and Performance Training*, 11 (1): 25–39.

Camilleri, Frank. 2020b. 'A Hybridity Continuum: The Case of the Performer's Bodyworlds', *Performance Research*, 25 (4): 17–25.

Camilleri, Frank. [2020] 2022. 'Of Assemblages, Affordances, and Actants – Or the Performer as Bodyworld: The Case of Puppet and Material Performance', *Studies in Theatre and Performance*, 42 (2): 156–69.

Camilleri, Frank. 2023. 'Seeing it Feelingly: On Affect and Bodyworld in Performance', *New Theatre Quarterly*, 39 (1): 69–80.

Camilleri, Frank, and John J. Schranz. 1996. *Id-Descartes: Identity of a Dramaturgy* (Malta: Groups for Human Encounter).

Cappuccio, Massimiliano L. 2019. 'Introduction', in Massimiliano L. Cappuccio (ed.), *Handbook of Embodied Cognition and Sport Psychology* (Cambridge, MA: MIT Press), pp. xv–xxxv.

Cappuccio, Massimiliano L., Rob Gray, Denise M. Hill, Christopher Mesagno, and Thomas H. Carr. 2019. 'The Many Threats of Self-Consciousness: Embodied Approaches to Choking under Pressure in Sensorimotor Skills', in Massimiliano L. Cappuccio (ed.), *Handbook of Embodied Cognition and Sport Psychology* (Cambridge, MA: MIT Press), pp. 101–55.

Carreri, Roberta. 2003. 'A Handful of Characters', *Open Page: Theatre – Women – Character*, 8: 44–54.

Carreri, Roberta. 2014. *On Training and Performance: Traces of an Odin Teatret Actress*, trans. by Frank Camilleri (London: Routledge).

Christensen, Wayne, and Kath Bicknell. 2019. 'Affordances and the Anticipatory Control of Action', in Massimiliano L. Cappuccio (ed.), *Handbook of Embodied Cognition and Sport Psychology* (Cambridge, MA: MIT Press), pp. 601–21.

Colombetti, Giovanna. 2014. *The Feeling Body: Affective Science Meets the Enactive Mind* (London: The MIT Press).

Colombetti, Giovanna. 2017. 'Enactive Affectivity, Extended', *Topoi*, 36 (3): 445–55.

Creely, Edwin. 2010. 'Method(ology), Pedagogy and Praxis: A Phenomenology of the Pre-Performative Training Regime of Phillip Zarrilli', *Theatre, Dance and Performance Training*, 1 (2): 214–28.

Cregan-Reid, Vybarr. 2016. *Footnotes: How Running Makes Us Human* (London: Ebury Press).

Csikszentmihalyi, Mihaly. 1990. *Flow: The Psychology of Optimal Experience* (New York: Harper Perennial).

Csikszentmihalyi, Mihaly. 1996. *Creativity: Flow and The Psychology of Discovery and Invention* (New York: Harper Perennial).

186 *References*

Csikszentmihalyi, Mihaly, and Isabela Selega Csikszentmihalyi (eds). 1988. *Optimal Experience; Psychological Studies of Flow in Consciousness* (Cambridge: Cambridge University Press).

Decroux, Étienne. [1963] 1985. *Words on Mime*, trans. by Mark Piper (Claremont, CA: Mime Journal).

Derrida, Jacques. [1967] 1978. 'The Theater of Cruelty and the Closure of Representation', in *Writing and Difference*, trans. by Alan Bass (London: Routledge), pp. 232–50.

Dewey, John. [1934] 1980. *Art as Experience* (New York: Perigee).

Dewsbury, John-David. 2012. 'Affective Habit Ecologies: Material Dispositions and Immanent Inhabitations', *Performance Research*, 17 (4): 74–82.

Dietrich, Arie, and W. F. McDaniel. 2004. 'Endocannabinoids and Exercise', *British Journal of Sports Medicine*, 38 (5): 536–41.

Duke, Robert A., Carla Davis Cash, and Sarah E. Allen. 2011. 'Focus of Attention Affects Performance of Motor Skills in Music', *Journal of Research in Music Education*, 59 (1): 44–55.

Duncan, Margot. 2004. 'Autoethnography: Critical Appreciation of an Emerging Art', *International Journal of Qualitative Methods*, 3 (4): 28–39.

Evans, Mark. 2012a. 'The Influence of Sports on Jacques Lecoq's Actor Training', *Theatre, Dance and Performance Training*, 3 (2): 163–77.

Evans, Mark. 2012b. 'Interview with Frantic Assembly: *Beautiful Burnout* and Training the Performer', *Theatre, Dance and Performance Training*, 3 (2): 258–68.

Evans, Mark. 2016. 'The Influence of Sports on Jacques Lecoq's Actor Training', in Mark Evans and Rick Kemp (eds), *The Routledge Companion to Jacques Lecoq* (London: Routledge), pp. 104–11.

Evans, Mark, and Simon Murray. 2012. 'Editorial', *Theatre, Dance and Performance Training*, 3 (2): 141–4.

Fitzgerald, Matt. 2016. *How Bad Do You Want It? Mastering the Psychology of Mind over Muscle* (London: Aurum Press).

Ford, Richard R., and Donna O'Connor. 2019. 'Practice and Sports Activities in the Acquisition of Anticipation and Decision Making', in A. Mark Williams and Robin C. Jackson (eds), *Anticipation and Decision Making in Sport* (London: Routledge), pp. 270–85.

Fortier, Mark. 2016. *Theory/Theatre: An Introduction*, 3rd edn (London: Routledge).

Gallagher, Shaun, and Julia Gallagher. 2020. 'Acting Oneself as Another: An Actor's Empathy for her Character', *Topoi*, 39 (1): 779–90.

Garmin. 2022. https://connect.garmin.com/modern/ (accessed 24 August 2022).

Geertz, Clifford. 1973. 'Thick Description: Toward an Interpretive Theory of Culture', in *The Interpretation of Cultures: Selected Essays* (New York: Basic Books, 1973), pp. 3–30.

Gibson, James J. [1979] 2015. *The Ecological Approach to Visual Perception* (London: Routledge).

Goodall, Jane. 2008. *Stage Presence* (London: Routledge).

Gray, Rob. 2015. 'Movement Automaticity in Sport', in Joseph Baker and Damian Farrow (eds), *Routledge Handbook of Sport Expertise* (London: Routledge), pp. 74–83.

Gregg, Melissa, and Gregory J. Seigworth (eds). 2010. *The Affect Theory Reader* (Durham, NC: Duke University Press).

Grotowski, Jerzy. [1968] 2002. *Towards a Poor Theatre* (London: Routledge).

Grotowski, Jerzy. 2006. 'Pragmatic Laws', in Eugenio Barba and Nicola Savarese (eds), *A Dictionary of Theatre Anthropology: The Secret Art of the Performer*, 2nd edn (London: Routledge), pp. 268–9.

Halperin, Israel, and Andrew D. Vigotsky. 2016. 'The Mind–Muscle Connection in Resistance Training: Friend or Foe?', *European Journal of Applied Physiology*, 116: 863–4.

Hill, Archibald Vivian, Cyril Norman Hugh Long, and H. Lupton. 1924. 'Muscular Exercise, Lactic Acid and the Supply and Utilisation of Oxygen. Parts VII – VIII', *Proceedings of the Royal Society London B*, 97: 155–76.

Hockey, John. 2013. 'Knowing the "Going": The Sensory Evaluation of Distance Running', *Qualitative Research in Sport, Exercise and Health*, 5 (1): 127–41.

Hodge, Alison (ed.). 2010a. *Actor Training*, 2nd edn (London: Routledge).

Hodge, Alison. 2010b. 'Włodzimierz Staniewski: Gardzienice and the Naturalised Actor', in Alison Hodge (ed.), *Actor Training*, 2nd edn (London: Routledge), pp. 269–87.

Hogan, Patrick Colm. 2016. 'Affect Studies', *Oxford Research Encyclopedias*. https://doi.org/10.1093/acrefore/9780190201098.013.105 (accessed 24 August 2022).

Hutchinson, Alex. 2018. *Endure: Mind, Body, and the Curiously Elastic Limits of Human Performance* (London: Harper Collins).

Icarus Performance Project. 2022. www.icarusproject.info (accessed 24 August 2022).

Ihde, Don. 1990. *Technology and the Lifeworld: From Garden to Earth* (Bloomington: Indiana University Press).

Jackson, Susan A. 1996. 'Toward a Conceptual Understanding of the Flow Experience in Elite Athletes', *Research Quarterly for Exercise and Sport*, 67 (1): 76–90.

Jackson, Susan A., and Mihaly Csikszentmihalyi. 1999. *Flow in Sports: The Keys to Optimal Experiences and Performances* (Champaign, IL: Human Kinetics).

Kapsali, Maria. 2021. *Performer Training and Technology* (London: Routledge).

Kirsh, David, and Paul Maglio. 1994. 'On Distinguishing Epistemic from Pragmatic Action', *Cognitive Science*, 18 (4): 513–49.

Krutak, Lars. 2014. '(Sur)real or Unreal? Antonin Artaud in the Sierra Tarahumara of Mexico', *Journal of Surrealism and the Americas*, 8 (1): 28–50.

Laban, Rudolf. [1939] 1966. *Choreutics*, annotated and edited by Lisa Ullmann (London: MacDonald and Evans).

188 *References*

Land, William Marshall. 2007. 'Facilitation of Automaticity: Sport-Relevant vs. Non-Relevant Secondary Tasks' (unpublished MSc thesis, Florida State University). https://diginole.lib.fsu.edu/islandora/object/fsu:181626/datastream/PDF/view (accessed 24 August 2022).

Land, William Marshall, and Gershon Tenenbaum. 2007. 'Facilitation of Automaticity: Sport-Relevant vs. Non-Relevant Secondary Tasks', presented at the North American Society for the Psychology of Sport and Physical Activity (NASPSPA), San Diego, California (2007), *Journal of Sport and Exercise Psychology*, 29 (s178).

Laster, Dominika. 2012. 'Embodied Memory: Body-Memory in the Performance Research of Jerzy Grotowski', *New Theatre Quarterly*, 28 (3): 211–29.

Latour, Bruno. 2005. *Reassembling the Social: An Introduction to Actor-Network-Theory* (Oxford: Oxford University Press).

Leabhart, Thomas. 1989. *Modern and Post-Modern Mime* (London: Macmillan).

Leabhart, Thomas. 1996. 'L'Homme de Sport: Sport, Statuary and the Recovery of the Pre-Cartesian Body in Etienne Decroux's Corporeal Mime', *Mime Journal: Theatre and Sport*, 31–65.

Leabhart, Thomas. 2022. *Copeau/Decroux, Irving/Craig: A Search for 20th Century Mime, Mask & Marionette* (London: Routledge).

Leabhart, Thomas, and Franc Chamberlain (eds). 2008. *The Decroux Sourcebook* (London: Routledge).

Lecoq, Jacques. [1997] 2002. *The Moving Body: Teaching Creative Theatre*, rev. edn, trans. by David Bradby (London: Bloomsbury).

Lecoq, Jacques. [1987] 2006. *Theatre of Movement and Gesture*, trans. and edited by David Bradby (London: Routledge).

Leeder, Jonathan, Conor Gissane, Ken van Someren, Warren Gregson, and Glyn Howatson. 2012. 'Cold Water Immersion and Recovery from Strenuous Exercise: A Meta-Analysis', *British Journal of Sports Medicine*, 46 (4): 233–40.

Lehmann, Hans-Thies. 2006. *Postdramatic Theatre*, trans. by Karen Jürs-Munby (London: Routledge).

Lennox, Solomon P. 2012. 'The Training of Boxer-Entertainers in Brendan Ingle's Gym', *Theatre, Dance and Performance Training*, 3 (2): 208–15.

Lennox, Solomon P., and George Rodosthenous. 2016. 'The Boxer–Trainer, Actor–Director Relationship: An Exploration of Creative Freedom', *Sport in Society*, 19 (2): 147–58.

Leys, Ruth. 2011. 'The Turn to Affect: A Critique', *Critical Inquiry*, 37 (3): 434–72.

Lindh, Ingemar. 1995. '"Gathering Around the Word Theatre ...", in Pentti Paavolainen and Anu Ala-Korpela (eds), *Knowledge is a Matter of Doing* (Helsinki: Acta Scenica), pp. 58–80.

Lindh, Ingemar. 2010. *Stepping Stones* (Abingdon: Routledge Icarus).

References 189

Liu, Zuo-Liang, Wing-Kai Lam, Xianyi Zhang, Benedicte Vanwanseele, and Hui Liu. 2021. 'Influence of Heel Design on Lower Extremity Biomechanics and Comfort Perception in Overground Running', *Journal of Sports Sciences*, 39 (2): 232–8.

Loukes, Rebecca. 2013. 'Beyond the Psychophysical? The "Situated", "Enactive" Bodymind in Performance', in Phillip B. Zarrilli, Jerry Daboo, and Rebecca Loukes, *Acting: Psychophysical Phenomenon and Process* (Houndmills: Palgrave Macmillan), pp. 224–55.

Lyotard, Jean-François. 1984. 'Answering the Question: What is Postmodernism?' trans. by Régis Durand, appendix in Jean-François Lyotard, *The Postmodern Condition: A Report on Knowledge*, trans. by Geoff Bennington and Brain Massumi (Minneapolis: University of Minnesota Press), pp. 71–82.

MacIntyre, Tadhg E., Christopher R. Madan, Noel E. Brick, Jürgen Beckmann, and Aidan P. Moran. 2019. 'Imagery, Expertise, and Action: A Window into Embodiment', in Massimiliano L. Cappuccio (ed.), *Handbook of Embodied Cognition and Sport Psychology* (Cambridge, MA: MIT Press), pp. 625–50.

Maldonato, Nelson Mauro, Alberto Oliverio, and Anna Esposito. 2019. 'Prefiguration, Anticipation, and Improvisation: A Neurocognitive and Phenomenological Perspective', in Massimiliano L. Cappuccio (ed.), *Handbook of Embodied Cognition and Sport Psychology* (Cambridge, MA: MIT Press), pp. 695–721.

Marcora, Samuele M. 2008. 'Do We Really Need a Central Governor to Explain Brain Regulation of Exercise Performance?', *European Journal of Applied Physiology*, 104 (5): 929–31.

Marcora, Samuele M. 2009. 'Perception of Effort during Exercise is Independent of Afferent Feedback from Skeletal Muscles, Heart, and Lungs', *European Journal of Applied Physiology*, 106 (6): 2060–2.

Marcora, Samuele. 2022. Personal profile page, University of Kent (UK). https://www.kent.ac.uk/sport-sciences/people/2189/marcora-samuele (accessed 24 August 2022).

Massumi, Brian. 2002. *Parables for the Virtual: Movement, Affect, Sensation* (Durham, NC: Duke University Press).

McDougall, Christopher. 2010. *Born to Run: The Hidden Tribe, the Ultra-Runners, and the Greatest Race the World Has Never Seen* (London: Profile Books).

Moran, Aidan. 2012. 'Thinking in Action: Some Insights from Cognitive Sport Psychology', *Thinking Skills and Creativity*, 7 (2): 85–92.

Morgan, William P., and Michael L. Pollock. 1977. 'Psychologic Characterization of the Elite Distance Runner', *Annals of the New York Academy of Sciences*, 301 (1): 382–403.

Murakami, Haruki. 2008. *What I Talk About When I Talk About Running* (London: Vintage).

Murphy, Maiya. 2019a. *Enacting Lecoq: Movement in Theatre, Cognition, and Life* (London: Palgrave Macmillan).

Murphy, Maiya. 2019b. '"Moritz to Fritz" A Response to *Performer Training Reconfigured: Post-Psychophysical Perspectives for the Twenty-First Century* by Frank Camilleri', *Theatre, Dance and Performance Training Blog*. 24 September. http://theatredanceperformancetraining.org/2019/09/moritz-to-fritz-a-response-to-performer-training-reconfigured-post-psychophysical-perspectives-for-the-twenty-first-century-by-frank-camilleri/ (accessed 24 August 2022).

Murray, Simon. 2003. *Jacques Lecoq* (London: Routledge).

Murray, Simon, and John Keefe. 2016. *Physical Theatres: A Critical Introduction*, 2nd edn (London: Routledge).

Nelson, Robin. 2013. *Practice as Research in the Arts: Principles, Protocols, Pedagogies, Resistances* (Houndmills: Palgrave Macmillan).

Nietfeld, John. 2003. 'An Examination of Metacognitive Strategy Use and Monitoring Skills by Competitive Middle Distance Runners', *Journal of Applied Sport Psychology*, 15 (4): 307–20.

Noakes, Timothy David, Juha E. Peltonen, and Heikke K. Rusko. 2001. 'Evidence that a Central Governor Regulates Exercise Performance during Acute Hypoxia and Hyperoxia', *Journal of Experimental Biology*, 204 (18): 3225–34.

Noakes, Timothy David, Alan St Clair Gibson, and Estelle Victoria Lambert. 2004. 'From Catastrophe to Complexity: A Novel Model of Integrative Central Neural Regulation of Effort and Fatigue during Exercise in Humans', *British Journal of Sports Medicine*, 38 (4): 511–14.

Noakes, Timothy David, Alan St Clair Gibson, and Estelle Victoria Lambert. 2005. 'From Catastrophe to Complexity: A Novel Model of Integrative Central Neural Regulation of Effort and Fatigue during Exercise in Humans: Summary and Conclusions', *British Journal of Sports Medicine*, 39 (2): 120–4.

Noakes, Timothy David, and Ross Tucker. 2008. 'Do We Really Need a Central Governor to Explain Brain Regulation of Exercise Performance? A Response to the Letter of Dr. Marcora', *European Journal of Applied Physiology*, 104 (5): 933–5.

O'Regan, J. Kevin, and Alva Noë. 2001. 'A Sensorimotor Approach to Vision and Visual Consciousness', *Behavioral and Brain Sciences*, 24 (5): 939–73.

Papoulias, Constantina, and Felicity Callard. 2010. 'Biology's Gift: Interrogating the Turn to Affect', *Body & Society*, 16 (1): 29–56.

Pasley, James. 2019. 'Inside Kenya's Rift Valley, which Produces the World's Best Marathon Runners Year after Year', *Insider*. 9 November. https://www.businessinsider.com/rift-valley-kenya-training-ground-world-best-runners-2019-11 (accessed 24 August 2022).

Patania, Vittoria Maria, Johnny Padulo, Enzo Iuliano, Luca Paolo Ardigò, Dražen Čular, Alen Miletić, and Andrea De Giorgio. 2020. 'The

Psychophysiological Effects of Different Tempo Music on Endurance versus High-Intensity Performances', *Frontiers in Psychology*, 11 (article 74): 1–7.

Porter, Jared M., Philip M. Anton, and Will F. W. Wu. 2012. 'Increasing the Distance of an External Focus of Attention Enhances Standing Long Jump Performance', *Journal of Strength and Conditioning Research*, 26 (9): 2389–93.

Quintana, Miguel, Oswaldo Rivera, Ricardo De La Vega, and Roberto Ruiz. 2012. 'Mapping the Runner's Mind: A New Methodology for Real-Time Tracking of Cognitions', *Psychology*, 3 (8): 590–4.

Rebellato, Dan. 2010. 'Katie Mitchell: Learning from Europe', in Maria M. Delgado and Dan Rebellato (eds), *Contemporary European Theatre Directors* (London: Routledge), pp. 317–38.

Richards, Thomas. 1995. *At Work with Grotowski on Physical Actions* (London: Routledge).

Ridout, Nicolas. 2006. *Stage Fright, Animals, and Other Theatrical Problems* (Cambridge: Cambridge University Press).

Roach, Joseph. 2007. *It* (Ann Arbor, MI: University of Michigan Press).

Robertson, Andy. 2020. 'With Andy Robertson', *That Peter Crouch Podcast*, BBC Radio 5 Live, 7 May 2020. https://www.bbc.co.uk/programmes/p08clwgm (accessed 24 August 2022).

Rodenburg, Patsy. 1992. *The Right to Speak: Working with the Voice* (London: Methuen).

Ruffini, Franco. 1995. 'Mime, The Actor, Action: The Way of Boxing', trans. by David Salgarolo, *Mime Journal: Incorporated Knowledge*, 54–69.

Ruffini, Franco. 2014. *Theatre and Boxing: The Actor Who Flies*, trans. by Paul Warrington (Holstebro, Malta, and Wrocław: Routledge Icarus).

Sander, David, and Klaus R. Scherer (eds). 2009. *The Oxford Companion to Emotion and the Affective Sciences* (Oxford: Oxford University Press).

Schatzki, Theodore R. 2001. 'Introduction: Practice Theory', in Theodore R. Schatzki, Karin Knorr-Cetina, and Eike Von Savigny (eds), *The Practice Turn in Contemporary Theory* (London: Routledge), pp. 1–14.

Schatzki, Theodore R., Karin Knorr-Cetina, and Eike Von Savigny (eds). 2001. *The Practice Turn in Contemporary Theory* (London: Routledge).

Schechner, Richard. 2013. *Performance Studies: An Introduction*, 3rd edn (London: Routledge).

Schino, Mirella. 2009. *Alchemists of the Stage: Theatre Laboratories in Europe*, trans. by Paul Warrington (Holstebro, Malta, and Wrocław: Routledge Icarus).

Schoenfeld, Brad J., and Bret Contreras. 2016. 'Attentional Focus for Maximizing Muscle Development: The Mind-Muscle Connection', *Strength and Conditioning Journal*, 38 (1): 27–9.

Selioni, Kiki. 2022. 'The Makings of the Actor'. https://themakingsactor.com/ (accessed 24 August 2022).

References

Shapiro, Lawrence, and Shannon Spaulding. 2019. 'Embodied Cognition and Sport', in Massimiliano L. Cappuccio (ed.), *Handbook of Embodied Cognition and Sport Psychology* (Cambridge, MA: MIT Press), pp. 3–21.

Shepherd, Simon, and Mick Wallis. 2004. *Drama/Theatre/Performance* (London: Routledge).

Shevtsova, Maria, and Christopher Innes. 2009. *Directors/Directing: Conversations on Theatre* (Cambridge: Cambridge University Press).

Shouse, Eric. 2005. 'Feeling, Emotion, Affect', *M/C Journal* 8 (6). https://doi.org/10.5204/mcj.2443 (accessed 24 August 2022).

Slowiak, James, and Jairo Cuesta. 2007. *Jerzy Grotowski* (London: Routledge).

Smith, Hazel, and Roger T. Dean (eds). 2010. *Practice-led Research, Research-led Practice in the Creative Arts* (Edinburgh: Edinburgh University Press).

Sokolicek, Alexander, Elizabeth R. Gebhard, and Rune Frederiksen (eds). 2015. *The Architecture of the Ancient Greek Theatre* (Aarhus: Aarhus University Press).

Soum, Corinne. 1997. 'Decroux the Ungraspable: Or Different Categories of Acting – Man of Sport, Man in the Drawing Room, Mobile Statuary, Man of Reverie', trans. by Thomas Leabhart, *Mime Journal: Words on Decroux 2*, 14–23.

Spearman, Peter. 2020. 'More Books', *TDR/The Drama Review*, 64 (2): 185–7.

Stanislavski, Constantin. [1936] 1989. *An Actor Prepares*, trans. by Elizabeth Reynolds Hapgood (London: Routledge).

Stanislavski, Konstantin. 2008. *An Actor's Work: A Student's Diary*, trans. and edited by Jean Benedetti (London: Routledge).

Steffen, Patrick. 2012. 'Forti on All Fours: A Talk with Simone Forti', *Contact Quarterly Online Journal* 37 (1). 9 January. https://contactquarterly.com/cq/unbound/index.php#view=onallfours. (accessed 24 August 2022).

Stevinson, Clare D., and Stuart J. H. Biddle. 1998. 'Cognitive Orientations in Marathon Running and "Hitting the Wall"', *British Journal of Sports Medicine*, 32 (3): 229–35.

Toner, John, and Barbara Montero. 2020. 'The Value of Aesthetic Judgements in Athletic Performance', *Journal of Somaesthetics*, 6 (1): 112–26.

Tucker, Ross. 2009. 'The Anticipatory Regulation of Performance: The Physiological Basis for Pacing Strategies and the Development of a Perception-based Model for Exercise Performance', *British Journal of Sports Medicine*, 43 (6): 392–400.

Turner, Bryan (ed.). 2012. *Routledge Handbook of Body Studies* (London: Routledge).

Turner, Bryan. 2012. 'Introduction: The Turn of the Body', in Bryan Turner (ed.), *Routledge Handbook of Body Studies* (London: Routledge), pp. 1–17.

Utterback, Neal. 2016. 'The Olympic Actor: Improving Actor Training and Performance through Sports Psychology', in Rhonda Blair and Amy Cook (eds), *Theatre, Performance and Cognition: Languages, Bodies and Ecologies* (London: Bloomsbury Methuen Drama), pp. 79–92.

References 193

Varley, Julia. [1995] 2021. 'Score and Sub-Score: A Useful but Wrong Word', *Journal of Theatre Anthropology*, 1: 213–20.

Wangh, Stephen. 2000. *An Acrobat of the Heart: A Physical Approach to Acting Inspired by the Work of Jerzy Grotowski* (New York: Vintage Books).

Watson, Ian. 2002. 'The Dynamics of Barter', in Ian Watson (ed.), *Negotiating Cultures: Eugenio Barba and the Intercultural Debate* (Manchester: Manchester University Press), pp. 94–111.

Whitehead, Patrick M. 2016. 'The Runner's High Revisited: A Phenomenological Analysis', *Journal of Phenomenological Psychology*, 47 (2): 183–98.

Whyman, Rose. 2013. *Stanislavski: The Basics* (London: Routledge).

Williams, A. Mark, and Robin C. Jackson (eds). 2019. *Anticipation and Decision Making in Sport* (London: Routledge).

Williams, Nerys. 2017. 'The Borg Rating of Perceived Exertion (RPE) scale', *Occupational Medicine*, 67 (5): 404–5.

Wilson, Andrew D., Qin Zhu, and Geoffrey P. Bingham. 2019. 'Affordances and the Ecological Approach to Throwing for Long Distances and Accuracy', in Massimiliano L. Cappuccio (ed.), *Handbook of Embodied Cognition and Sport Psychology* (Cambridge, MA: MIT Press), pp. 581–600.

Wolford, Lisa. 1997. 'General Introduction: Ariadne's Thread', in Richard Schechner and Lisa Wolford (eds), *The Grotowski Sourcebook* (London: Routledge), pp. 1–18.

Worth, Libby (ed.). 2015. Special issue, 'Moshe Feldenkrais', *Theatre, Dance and Performance Training*, 6 (2).

Wulf, Gabriele. 2008. 'Attentional Focus Effects in Balance Acrobats', *Research Quarterly for Exercise and Sport*, 79 (3): 319–25.

Wulf, Gabriele. 2013. 'Attentional Focus and Motor Learning: A Review of 15 Years', *International Review of Sport and Exercise Psychology*, 6 (1): 77–104.

Wulf, Gabriele, Markus Höß, and Wolfgang Prinz. 1998. 'Instructions for Motor Learning: Differential Effects of Internal versus External Focus of Attention', *Journal of Motor Behavior*, 30 (2): 169–79.

Wulf, Gabriele, Nancy McNevin, and Charles H. Shea. 2001. 'The Automaticity of Complex Motor Skill Learning as a Function of Attentional Focus', *Quarterly Journal of Experimental Psychology*, 54 (4): 1143–54.

Wulf, Gabriele, and Rebecca Lewthwaite. 2010. 'Effortless Motor Learning? An External Focus of Attention Enhances Movement Effectiveness and Efficiency', in Brian Bruya (ed.), *Effortless Attention: A New Perspective in the Cognitive Science of Attention and Action* (Cambridge, MA: MIT Press), pp. 75–101.

Zarrilli, Phillip B. 2004. 'Toward a Phenomenological Model of the Actor's Embodied Modes of Experience', *Theatre Journal*, 56 (4): 653–66.

Zarrilli, Phillip B. 2009. *Psychophysical Acting: An Intercultural Approach after Stanislavski* (London: Routledge).

194   *References*

Zarrilli, Phillip B. 2010. 'Religious and Civic Festivals: Early Drama and Theatre in Context', in Gary Jay Williams (ed.), *Theatre Histories: An Introduction*, 2nd edn (London: Routledge), pp. 52–88.

Zarrilli, Phillip B. 2013. 'Introduction: Acting as Psychophysical Phenomenon and Process', in Phillip B. Zarrilli, Jerry Daboo, and Rebecca Loukes, *Acting: Psychophysical Phenomenon and Process* (Houndmills: Palgrave Macmillan), pp. 1–50.

Zarrilli, Phillip B. 2020. *(Toward) A Phenomenology of Acting* (London: Routledge).

Index

acrobatics, acrobats 16–18, 24, 50, 55, 60, 74

actant 4–5, 27, 58, 109, 176

affect (*see also* intensities) xxii, 16–17, 102–5, 112–13, 116, 156, 171

affective science 102–4, 106–7, 112, 121, 131

affect theory 102–4, 115, 121, 131

affordances xx, xxv, 4–5, 9–14, 16, 19–20, 27, 57–58, 108–9, 115, 124, 169–70, 175–6

agency 5, 30, 76, 87, 141

agential realism xiii

Alexander Technique 47, 48, 54

Artaud, Antonin 15–18, 28
    affective athleticism xx, 16–17, 30

assemblage 4–5, 6, 9, 11, 33, 58, 83, 105, 108–9, 176

attentional focus 37–41, 44, 48, 53, 58, 61, 63, 68, 73–5, 97, 159, 176 *see also* cognition

automaticity xxi, 52, 58, 60, 64–5, 70–71, 80, 87, 91, 128, 163, 178

automatic pilot, autopilot 49–53

Barad, Karen xxv, 1–2

Barba, Eugenio (*see also* Odin Teatret) xiv, 42, 48, 62, 91–2, 125–8, 129, 152, 180

bodybuilding 22, 61

bodymind xiii, xxx, 2–4, 19, 39–42, 44–5, 68, 84, 98, 145

bodyworld xiii–xiv, xx–xxi, 2–5, 9, 14, 23, 30, 33, 38, 46–7, 83, 108–10, 141, 169–70

Borg, Gunnar 81, 84, 85

boxing 8, 15–16, 18, 21–7, 127, 168

breath 17, 34, 40–1, 47, 60, 94, 156, 159

Brick, Noel 37–41, 44, 50, 53, 85, 87, 138, 176

Carpentier, Georges 19, 21–4, 28

Carreri, Roberta xxi, 49–50, 52–3, 128–9, 180

central governor 79–82, 85–6, 127–8

Chekhov, Michael 129

choking xxviii, 65, 69–70, 113–14, 124, 163, 175–7

choreography 59, 67, 82, 91, 93, 97, 117, 130, 135, 178, 180 *see also* score

cognition (*see also* attentional focus; focus; monitoring) xix, xxi, 5, 33, 37, 39, 63, 133, 137, 140, 142–3, 155
    cognitive processing 37, 53, 67, 106, 122, 132, 137–41, 144, 150, 155, 175
    embodied cognition 9, 63, 79, 82–3, 164
    enactive cognition 3, 115
    enclothed cognition 108, 110
    metacognition 96, 124, 139, 144, 148

Colombetti, Giovanna 3, 112, 141

competitive, competitiveness xv, xx, 22, 61, 72, 112, 156–7
    collaborative competitiveness xxiv, 119, 169, 178
    hyper-competitiveness 22–3, 30

Copeau, Jacques 7, 18–20, 25–6, 29, 117

costume xxiii, xxix, 66–7, 108, 110–11

Cregan-Reid, Vybarr xix, 30, 37, 50, 109, 157

cross-training xvii, 47, 74, 179

Csikszentmihalyi, Mihaly 62–5, 161–3, 179

Decroux, Étienne 18–23, 25–7,
125–6, 169, 170
Homme de Sport (Man of Sport)
20
Derrida, Jacques 15
devising 147, 149, 173
Diderot, Denis 94
disabled, disability xxv, 1–2
distraction xxi, 37–8, 48–51, 53, 59,
62, 64, 71, 76, 87, 138, 154,
163, 176, 179
dynamic aliveness 147, 152–61,
163–4, 168, 179, 180

effort 13, 20, 21, 27, 36, 38, 46, 49–51,
53, 85, 87–9, 95, 106, 131, 153,
155, 172
perception of effort 49, 51, 71, 80,
85–6, 92–3, 98, 101, 105, 132,
139, 177
embodiment xviii, 1–3, 24, 38, 40, 53,
108, 137–8, 166, 181
emotion xx, xxii–xxiii, 9, 16–17, 21,
36, 94–5, 101–5, 111, 121–2,
129–31, 134, 137, 141, 143,
167–9, 172–3, 177
emotion episode 105–7, 114,
118–20, 137, 166
emotion modulation 106, 122,
131–3, 135
endurance xii, xix, 35, 38, 43, 49, 54,
81–5, 127, 140
endurance sports xxii, 9, 29–30,
37, 55, 79, 89, 93, 154, 169, 170
ensemble 89, 163
epistemic actions xxi, 27, 65–9, 71–2,
74, 139, 179
ethics 15, 21, 24–7, 28, 168, 169
exhaustion 35, 49, 51–3, 156, 160

Feldenkrais, Moshé 47, 48, 54
Fitzgerald, Matt 28, 29, 55, 84, 85, 88,
93, 96, 101–2, 105, 132, 170
flow xxi, 18, 35, 61–5, 69, 71, 77, 156,
161–4, 175, 178–9

focus (*see also* attentional focus) xxi,
xxviii, 38, 41, 51, 55, 70, 73,
97, 139, 153, 163
external focus 37, 58, 60–1, 63–4,
66, 74–5, 176
focused distraction 71–2, 87, 154,
158
internal focus 58–62, 65, 66, 75,
114, 124, 163, 175–6
football 48, 72, 76, 91, 97, 110,
118–19, 124, 126, 144, 162, 179
footwear xix, xxii, 11, 13, 66, 85,
108–9, 140, 175
Forti, Simone 3–4, 39

game, games (*see also* play) 8, 13, 61,
72, 91, 95, 97, 115–16, 118–19
Gibson, James J. 10–12
GPS fitness tracking xvi, xvii, 46,
50–51, 54
Grotowski, Jerzy xiv, 17, 28, 29, 35,
40, 129–30, 154, 165

habit 25, 48–9, 50, 59, 70, 108, 115
habitational action xxx, 90, 108,
138, 141, 148, 165, 170–1,
178, 180
Hébert, Georges 18–20, 22, 30, 169
auto-émulation 20, 22 169
Hogan, Patrick Colm xxii, 103, 104,
106–7, 112, 119, 122, 131, 137,
139–40, 156
Hutchinson, Alex 46, 80, 85–6, 88, 128

Icarus Performance Project (Malta)
xiv, 150, 157, 171, 174 *see also*
Martyr Red
Id-Descartes xxv, 157–8
Ihde, Don 3
imagination 26, 30, 40, 59–60, 63, 72,
75, 87, 95, 148, 149, 162, 164,
172, 177
improvisation xvi, xxiii, xxiv, 63,
90–1, 93, 117–19, 145, 147–51,
157, 160, 161–5, 171, 178

collective improvisation 123, 134, 163, 174
Ingle, Brandon 23–27, 168
intensities (*see also* affect) 103, 105, 107, 109, 111, 116, 119
intentionality xviii, 12–14, 40, 59, 76, 124–5, 127–30, 148–9, 172, 173, 179, 180
invisible dimension xiv–xvii, 6
isometric exercises 122–5

Keigo 1–2, 3, 27, 30

Laban, Rudolf 74, 174
Leabhart, Thomas 18, 20, 21
Lecoq, Jacques 20, 25–6, 34, 110, 117–19, 141–3, 164, 169
Lennox, Solomon P. 23–4
lifeworld 3
Lindh, Ingemar xiv, 29, 35, 87, 123–4, 126, 134–5, 150, 170, 174, 179–80
Loukes, Rebecca 67–8, 179

marathon, half-marathon, ultramarathon xvi–xvii, xxx, 4, 33, 37, 43, 45, 52, 54, 86, 109, 139–40, 153, 181
Marcora, Samuele xxii, 83, 84–6, 122, 139
martial arts 8, 16, 47, 55, 67, 74, 98, 150
Martyr Red 157, 159–60
McDougall, Christopher xix, 15, 109
mask 20, 109–10, 117, 164, 165
Massumi, Brian 102–5, 113, 119, 132, 137, 140
metacognitive *see under* cognition
mime 18–19, 20, 21, 29, 34, 125, 126, 142, 143, 169, 170
mindfulness 71, 74, 84
mind–muscle connection 58, 60
Mitchell, Katie 124
monitoring (outward, internal/sensory) xvi, 37–8, 40,

44–6, 58, 63, 87–9, 91, 98, 106, 138, 154, 176, 177 *see also* cognition
Murakami, Haruki 33–6, 52–3, 57–8, 153
Murphy, Maiya 141–3, 164
music, musicians 8, 38, 61–3, 85, 91, 143, 147, 160, 162–4

Nelson, Robin 46, 138, 146, 160
neuroscience 39, 63, 79, 83, 161, 162
Noakes, Timothy 79–80, 82–3, 85–6, 92, 128, 144

Odin Teatret 7, 49, 50, 63, 69, 71, 91, 127, 128, 180
ontology xvi, 4, 18, 68, 69
O'Regan, J. Kevin 51–2, 115
organic 59, 73, 84, 92, 121, 147, 175

pacing and aesthetic pacing xvii, xxii, xxiv, xxx, 38, 79, 81–2, 87–9, 93–8, 105–6, 119, 145, 152, 154, 178–81
parkour 19
phenomenological tone 106–7, 122, 135, 137, 143, 145, 150, 152, 155–7, 161
phenomenology 62, 98, 109, 152–3
physical theatre 29, 34, 47, 67, 73, 80, 121, 157, 164, 171
plastiques 147, 149–53, 157, 159–61, 164, 174
play xv, xx, xiv, 13, 25–6, 117–19, 142, 163–4, 169, 170, 177, 178
post-psychophysical xi, 2–4, 44–5, 66, 141
postdramatic theatre 89
postphenomenology xiii, 3
posture 47, 54, 109, 126, 127, 135, 155
psychobiological 79, 82–4, 85, 122, 139
psychophysical xi, xiii, xvii, xxiv, 4, 7, 25, 38, 39, 44, 50, 55, 59,

70, 79–81, 83–4, 88, 97, 109, 125–7, 146, 162, 170, 174–6

Raczak, Lech xiv
rate of perceived effort (RPE) 80–2, 85, 95–6, 101, 106, 139, 144
regulation xxiii, 82, 104, 106, 131, 168, 177
    active self-regulation 37–38, 40, 42, 45, 46, 50–1, 87
    anticipatory regulation 79–81, 87, 92–3, 98, 144, 153
repetition xvi, xxviii, 49, 53, 61, 64, 91, 179
Richards, Thomas xxi, 7, 35, 40, 52–3
Ruffini, Franco 18–20, 22–6, 29, 148, 167–8, 180
running xv–xix, xxvii, xxix, 12, 19, 21, 30, 33–6, 38, 44, 46–8, 50, 54, 66, 91, 97, 105, 132, 139–41, 155, 157, 170
    long-distance running (*see also* marathon) xi–xii, 9, 43, 101, 152–5, 179
    runners xxii, 15, 16, 36, 38, 42, 44, 49, 58, 61, 80, 96, 108, 110, 144, 146, 167, 168, 181

sailing 10, 12
sats xxiii, 91, 125–9
Schranz, John J. xiv, 154, 157, 174
score (performance) 36, 42, 59, 63, 67, 70–1, 75, 91–4, 95–6, 117, 118, 148, 157–8, 160, 164–6, 178, 180, 181 *see also* choreography
secondary tasks xxi, 66, 68–73, 179
sensation xxii, 15, 36, 38, 39, 46, 50, 81, 84, 87, 102–7, 113–14, 129, 130, 133, 141, 143–5,
sensorimotor 9, 39, 69, 70, 116
    contingencies 51–2, 115
    exigencies 51, 52, 67, 73

shoes *see under* footwear
skilled behaviour 1, 9, 14, 24, 167, 181
sociomaterial xi, xiii, 103, 108
song, singing xxv, 8, 35, 73, 94, 158–9
Soum, Corinne 20, 21, 23
sphere exercise xxiv, 74–5, 171–4, 175–80
stage fright xxiii, xxviii, 65, 113–14, 133–4, 163, 176, 177
Stanislavski, Konstantin xii, 15, 17, 67–8, 76, 94–5, 111, 113–5, 124, 129, 133–4

technology xii–xiii, 1, 3, 4, 7, 11, 12, 36, 44–6, 50, 54, 109, 175 *see also* GPS fitness tracking
Tekhnē Sessions (see also Icarus Performance Project) 150–2, 157, 160, 161, 164
tennis 1, 91, 111–12, 113, 118, 127
theatricality 23–4, 26–7, 168
Tucker, Ross 80–2, 85–6, 106, 144

Varley, Julia 63–4, 66, 70–1, 75
via athletae xx, xxiv, xxv, xxxi, 14–18, 20–1, 23, 28–30, 90, 119, 167, 169–71, 174–81
visualization 37, 39, 41, 55, 59–60, 72, 171
voice, vocal (*see also* song) xxiv–xxvi, 7, 18, 49, 54, 59, 73, 75, 92, 94, 113, 118, 148, 150, 158–9, 173, 175

Wangh, Stephen 17–18
Wulf, Gabriele xxi, 42–3, 58–61, 64–6, 73–4, 97, 139, 176

yoga xvii, 18, 27, 47, 54, 55, 67, 147

Zarrilli, Phillip B. 3, 8, 38–43, 45, 47, 48, 55, 59, 60, 67, 84, 93, 98, 141, 145, 146, 152, 164

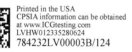
Printed in the USA
CPSIA information can be obtained
at www.ICGtesting.com
LVHW012335280624
784232LV00003B/124